Super Easy Anti-Infl

Diet Cookbook for Beginners:

2000 Days of Simple & Delicious Recipes with
a 30-Day Meal Plan
for Digestive Wellness and Weight Management.
Promote Wellness and Enjoy Healthy Living

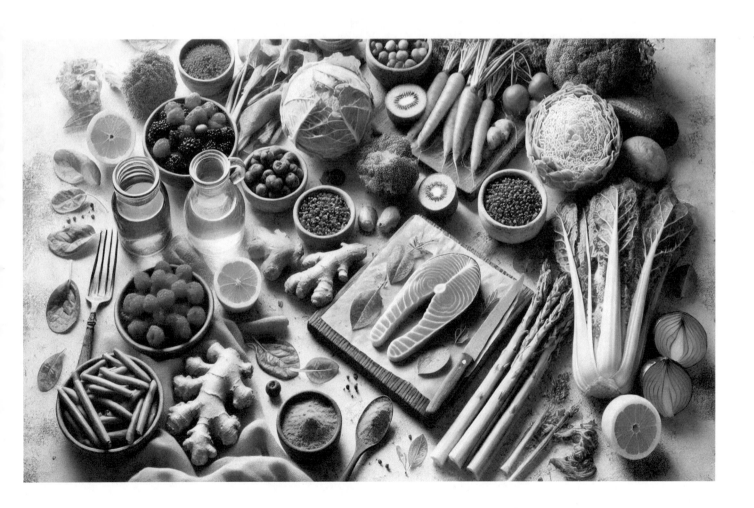

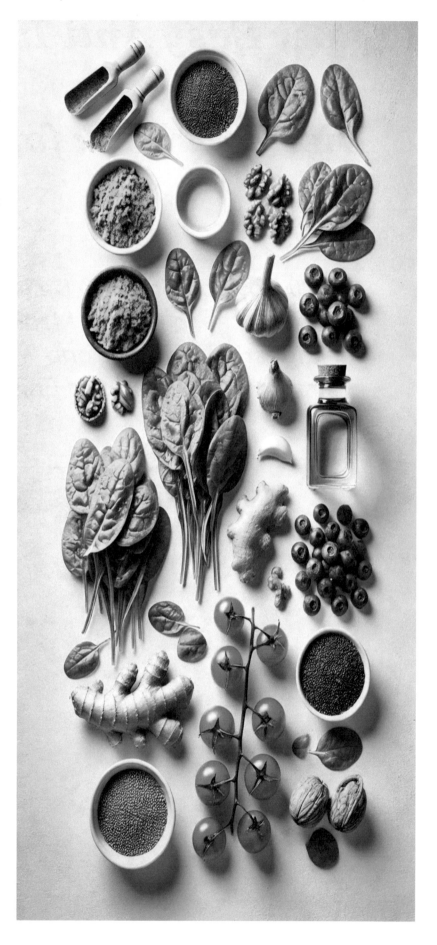

Table of Contents

INTRODUCTION

If you're reading this, chances are you're looking for a real, lasting way to improve your health. Whether you're battling a chronic condition like arthritis, diabetes, heart disease, or simply trying to regain control of your energy and weight, this is the first step toward meaningful change. It's not about drastic overhauls or quick fixes. It's about giving your body what it needs to naturally reduce inflammation and thrive.

For many of you, the idea of managing chronic symptoms without relying heavily on medication feels like a daunting challenge. The pain, the fatigue, the limitations—they all weigh heavily on your day-to-day life. But here's the good news: you have more control over your body's response to inflammation than you might think. A well-crafted, anti-inflammatory diet can be one of the most powerful tools in your toolkit, helping to alleviate symptoms, boost energy, and even prevent future health complications.

If you're someone who takes wellness seriously—whether through organic foods, fitness, or mindful eating—you're already ahead of the curve. This book is here to complement the practices you're already familiar with by offering easy, straightforward recipes that align with the latest health trends.

For those struggling with weight management, this book offers hope. Inflammation and weight gain are closely linked, and breaking the cycle starts with what you put on your plate. By eating in a way that naturally reduces inflammation, you'll likely see improvements not just in your waistline, but also in your energy levels, mood, and overall vitality.

Women, particularly those between 30 and 50, often face the unique challenges of balancing hormonal shifts, stress, and health concerns. This is a time when your body demands extra attention, and the foods you choose can make all the difference. Whether you're dealing with the effects of stress, hormone-related issues, or simply want to invest in long-term wellness, the recipes and tips in this book are designed with you in mind.

For our senior readers, managing inflammation is critical to maintaining mobility, reducing pain, and staying active. Joint pain, stiffness, and overall discomfort don't have to define your later years. By following an anti-inflammatory diet, you can experience a higher quality of life, with more freedom to do what you love.

Stress, for many of us, is an unavoidable part of life, and it's no secret that stress and inflammation feed off each other. One of the best ways to combat this vicious cycle is through your diet. The recipes in this book are not only designed to lower inflammation but also to help balance your body's response to stress. They are simple, quick, and perfect for those looking to make healthy changes without feeling overwhelmed.

So, where do you start? Right here, with the decision to take control of your health through small, consistent changes. This book will guide you, step by step, with recipes that are easy to follow, require no exotic ingredients, and fit seamlessly into your everyday routine. By focusing on whole, nutrient-rich foods, you'll begin to feel the difference in your body—less pain, more energy, and a clearer mind.

This journey is about more than just food. It's about adopting a mindset of wellness, taking small steps each day toward a healthier, happier life. You don't have to do it all at once—just start with one meal, one recipe, and see where it takes you. Your body will thank you.

CHAPTER 1: START HEALTHY NOW

Understand Inflammation

Inflammation is your body's natural defense mechanism. It's what happens when your immune system kicks into high gear to fight off infection, heal an injury, or defend against harmful invaders. However, when inflammation becomes chronic—constantly triggered by diet, stress, or lifestyle—it can turn from a helpful defense into a harmful force, contributing to diseases such as arthritis, diabetes, heart disease, and even autoimmune conditions.

For many of you, chronic inflammation has been a frustrating and exhausting part of your life. You might feel like you're constantly battling pain, fatigue, or discomfort with little relief. But here's the empowering truth: what you eat has a profound impact on this process. The food on your plate can either fuel the flames of inflammation or help extinguish them.

This book introduces you to the anti-inflammatory diet—a scientifically backed approach to nutrition that helps your body fight inflammation naturally. By choosing foods rich in antioxidants, healthy fats, and fiber while cutting out processed, sugary, and inflammatory foods, you'll take control of your body's response and start feeling the benefits quickly.

How This Diet Transforms You

The anti-inflammatory diet isn't just about treating symptoms; it's about creating a foundation for long-term health. One of the first things you'll notice is a shift in your energy levels. Chronic inflammation can zap your energy, making you feel sluggish and drained. As you start incorporating anti-inflammatory foods—like leafy greens, berries, fatty fish, and whole grains—you'll feel a noticeable boost in energy. Your body will spend less time fighting inflammation and more time thriving.

For those with conditions like arthritis or autoimmune disorders, reducing inflammation can mean less pain and better mobility. When you start fueling your body with foods that support healing rather than harm, you'll likely experience less stiffness, joint pain, and general discomfort. The impact goes beyond just physical relief—reducing inflammation can also improve your mood, sleep, and overall quality of life.

This diet also helps manage weight, which is crucial for many of you who are struggling with weight-related inflammation. Inflammation and weight gain often go hand in hand, creating a vicious cycle. By focusing on nutrient-dense, anti-inflammatory foods, you'll not only reduce inflammation but also support healthy, sustainable weight loss.

Unlock Gut Health and Weight Loss

Your gut plays a pivotal role in managing inflammation. An imbalanced gut, often caused by a diet high in processed foods, sugar, and unhealthy fats, can trigger inflammatory responses throughout the body. Improving your gut health is key to breaking the cycle of inflammation and unlocking the benefits of this diet.

Anti-inflammatory foods are naturally gut-friendly. They are rich in fiber, prebiotics, and probiotics, which help nourish the good bacteria in your digestive system. These foods help reduce bloating, promote regular digestion, and support a healthy balance of gut bacteria—all of which contribute to a stronger immune system and lower levels of inflammation.

As you improve your gut health, you'll likely notice changes in your waistline as well. A healthy gut improves your body's ability to metabolize food, stabilize blood sugar, and reduce cravings for unhealthy, inflammatory foods. This means easier, more sustainable weight management without restrictive dieting or deprivation.

By following the guidelines in this book, you'll begin to unlock the full potential of your body's natural healing powers—fighting inflammation at its source and transforming your health from the inside out.

Learn From Real Success Stories

There's something incredibly motivating about hearing real-life success stories, especially when it comes to making changes in your health. In this chapter, I want to share with you some of the remarkable transformations people have experienced by following an anti-inflammatory diet. These stories aren't just about weight loss or lowering numbers on a chart—they're about reclaiming a better quality of life, regaining mobility, and finding joy in everyday activities again.

Take Sarah, for example. At 42, she had been living with rheumatoid arthritis for over a decade. The pain and stiffness had become a constant presence in her life. She had tried medications, physical therapy, and various treatments, but nothing seemed to provide lasting relief. Frustrated with the side effects of medications, Sarah decided to take a more holistic approach and began incorporating an anti-inflammatory diet into her routine. Within weeks, she noticed a difference—not just in her pain levels but in her overall energy and mood. By

replacing processed foods and sugars with leafy greens, healthy fats, and antioxidant-rich fruits, Sarah found herself moving more freely, enjoying family activities, and, for the first time in years, waking up without pain.

Now, let's talk about Tom. At 55, Tom was diagnosed with Type 2 diabetes, and his doctor told him he needed to make serious changes. His blood sugar levels were high, his energy was low, and he was carrying extra weight, especially around his middle. Like many, Tom had tried restrictive diets in the past but couldn't stick with them. After discovering the anti-inflammatory diet, Tom didn't just focus on cutting calories—he focused on eating nutrient-dense, anti-inflammatory foods. He began including more fiber, whole grains, and healthy fats into his meals while reducing his intake of processed foods and refined carbs. Within six months, Tom's blood sugar levels had improved dramatically, his doctor reduced his medication, and he had lost over 20 pounds. More importantly, he felt energized and confident about maintaining this lifestyle for the long haul.

Discover Weight Loss and Gut Health Wins

Inflammation isn't just a problem for those with chronic illnesses—it's also a major barrier for people trying to lose weight. When your body is inflamed, it can affect your metabolism, making it harder to shed pounds even with a healthy diet and exercise. But as the success stories in this chapter show, once you reduce inflammation through diet, weight loss becomes a much more attainable goal.

Maria, a 38-year-old mother of two, struggled with her weight for years. She had tried every trendy diet—from low-carb to juice cleanses—but nothing seemed to stick. What Maria didn't realize was that her high-stress job and poor eating habits were causing chronic inflammation, which was sabotaging her weight loss efforts. When she switched to an anti-inflammatory diet, focusing on whole foods, lean proteins, and cutting out inflammatory triggers like sugar and processed snacks, the weight began to drop off. Maria lost 30 pounds in a year, but what was even more surprising was the improvement in her gut health. Her bloating disappeared, her digestion improved, and she finally felt comfortable in her own skin again. The combination of weight loss and improved gut health transformed Maria's life—not just physically, but mentally and emotionally as well.

Similarly, David, a 47-year-old businessman, was constantly on the go and often relied on fast food and caffeine to get through his busy days. Over time, his unhealthy eating habits caught up with him. David was dealing with frequent heartburn, digestive issues, and unwanted weight gain. After learning about the connection between gut health and inflammation, he decided to make a change. By prioritizing gut-friendly foods like fermented vegetables, fiber-rich grains, and lean proteins, David saw improvements not only in his digestion but also in his waistline. Within months, his digestion normalized, and he lost 25 pounds without feeling like he was on a diet. More importantly, his heartburn and digestive discomfort became a thing of the past.

Get Motivated by Real-Life Testimonials

What's so powerful about these stories is that they prove real change is possible, no matter what challenges you're facing. For people living with chronic conditions, it can feel like the deck is stacked against you. But as these stories show, making small, consistent changes to your diet can yield profound results. From reducing joint pain to improving energy, these individuals have not only transformed their health but also regained their confidence and independence. It's one thing to read about the benefits of an anti-inflammatory diet in theory—it's another to hear from real people who have walked this path before you. These testimonials are here to remind you that you're not alone in your journey, and success is not just possible—it's within reach.

So whether you're dealing with arthritis, diabetes, heart disease, or just looking to improve your overall well-being, take these stories as a source of inspiration. Let them remind you that change doesn't happen overnight, but with the right mindset and a commitment to better habits, you can achieve lasting health. And remember—your story could be the next one that inspires others to start their own journey.

Anti-Inflammatory Diet – Myths and Realities

The topic of inflammation has gained significant attention over the past few years, particularly when it comes to chronic diseases and overall well-being. While the idea of an anti-inflammatory diet is rooted in sound scientific principles, there are also a number of myths and misconceptions that have arisen. This chapter will break down the truth behind these claims and offer clarity on how an anti-inflammatory diet can truly benefit you.

Myth 1: Inflammation is Always Bad

It's important to understand that inflammation is a natural process that helps the body heal. When you cut yourself or catch a cold, your immune system activates to fight off infections and repair damaged tissue. In these cases, inflammation is necessary and beneficial. However, chronic inflammation – the kind that persists over time – is where problems begin. This type of inflammation can contribute to conditions like arthritis, heart disease, diabetes, and autoimmune disorders.

Reality: While inflammation is part of the body's defense system, chronic inflammation is harmful and can accelerate the aging process and lead to disease. The goal of an anti-inflammatory diet is not to eliminate inflammation entirely, but to manage it so that your body can function optimally without being in a constant state of repair.

Myth 2: The Anti-Inflammatory Diet is Only for People with Arthritis

The anti-inflammatory diet is often associated with managing joint pain, particularly in cases of arthritis. While it's true that certain foods can help reduce the severity of arthritis symptoms, the benefits of an anti-inflammatory diet extend far beyond this. Chronic inflammation is linked to a wide range of diseases, including cardiovascular disease, diabetes, and even mental health conditions like depression.

Reality: An anti-inflammatory diet benefits not only people with arthritis but also those looking to improve gut health, reduce cardiovascular risk, support metabolic health, and enhance overall well-being. It can help reduce systemic inflammation, benefiting people with a wide range of health concerns.

Myth 3: All Fats are Inflammatory

One of the most common myths about inflammation is that all fats are harmful. For years, people believed that reducing fat intake would automatically lead to better health. While trans fats and processed fats are indeed inflammatory, not all fats are created equal. Omega-3 fatty acids, which are found in foods like fatty fish, flaxseeds, and walnuts, actually help reduce inflammation.

Reality: Healthy fats are an essential part of an anti-inflammatory diet. Focus on incorporating sources of unsaturated fats, particularly omega-3s, which have been shown to reduce inflammation and promote heart health.

Myth 4: You Can't Have Carbs on an Anti-Inflammatory Diet

With the popularity of low-carb diets like keto, there is a widespread belief that carbohydrates are inherently bad and should be eliminated to reduce inflammation. However, this is a myth. Not all carbs are the same. Refined carbohydrates, such as white bread and pastries, can spike blood sugar and contribute to inflammation, but whole grains like quinoa, oats, and brown rice have anti-inflammatory properties.

Reality: Carbohydrates from whole food sources, such as fruits, vegetables, and whole grains, provide essential fiber and nutrients that support gut health and help reduce inflammation. The key is to choose complex, unprocessed carbs that provide long-lasting energy and support digestive health.

Myth 5: A Strict Diet is Required to See Results

There's a belief that you need to strictly adhere to a rigid set of dietary rules to see the benefits of an anti-inflammatory diet. While consistency is important, the good news is that you don't need to completely overhaul your diet overnight. Small, gradual changes can have a significant impact.

Reality: You don't have to give up all of your favorite foods. An anti-inflammatory diet is about balance. Focus on reducing your intake of processed foods, added sugars, and unhealthy fats while increasing your consumption of whole foods, vegetables, lean proteins, and healthy fats. Over time, you'll notice the benefits without feeling deprived.

Bringing it All Together

The reality of an anti-inflammatory diet is that it's a sustainable way to manage chronic inflammation and promote long-term health. There's no need for extreme measures or strict diets – it's about making informed choices that align with your health goals.

This approach is particularly beneficial for those with chronic conditions like arthritis, diabetes, or cardiovascular disease, but it's equally effective for anyone looking to boost their energy, improve gut health, and reduce the overall inflammatory burden on their body.

The anti-inflammatory diet is not a fad or a trend – it's a long-term, evidence-based approach to eating that empowers you to take control of your health, one meal at a time.

Mastering Meal Planning

Now that you have a solid understanding of the essential anti-inflammatory foods, it's time to put that knowledge into action by mastering meal planning. One of the keys to maintaining a healthy, anti-inflammatory diet is making sure that your meals are balanced, diverse, and enjoyable. The goal isn't to restrict yourself, but to create meals that nourish your body, reduce inflammation, and give you the energy you need to thrive.

In this chapter, we will dive into the practical aspects of meal planning, so you can confidently prepare delicious, anti-inflammatory meals for every day of the week.

1. The Importance of Meal Planning

Meal planning is more than just deciding what to eat. It's about being proactive in your approach to eating, ensuring that you always have nutritious, anti-inflammatory ingredients on hand and that your meals are balanced and satisfying. Meal planning can help you save time, reduce stress, and prevent the last-minute temptation of less healthy options.

Why it matters: When you plan your meals ahead of time, you're more likely to stick to your health goals, avoid processed foods, and enjoy meals that align with your anti-inflammatory diet. Planning also ensures that you're getting the right mix of macronutrients (proteins, healthy fats, and complex carbohydrates) and micronutrients (vitamins, minerals, and antioxidants).

2. Build Your Plate: The Anti-Inflammatory Formula

Every meal should aim to include a balance of the following:

Healthy fats: These could come from sources like olive oil, avocados, nuts, seeds, or fatty fish like salmon.

Lean protein: Include plant-based proteins like lentils, beans, or tofu, or lean animal proteins like chicken, turkey, or fish.

Colorful vegetables: At least half of your plate should be filled with a variety of vegetables, with an emphasis on leafy greens, cruciferous veggies (like broccoli and cauliflower), and brightly colored vegetables rich in antioxidants.

Whole grains: Opt for whole grains like quinoa, brown rice, farro, or barley. These provide fiber, essential for gut health and inflammation control.

Herbs and spices: Don't forget to add herbs like parsley, cilantro, and spices like turmeric, ginger, and garlic, all of which enhance the anti-inflammatory properties of your meals.

Why it matters: By following this simple formula, you ensure that each meal contains a variety of nutrients that will work together to reduce inflammation, support digestion, and maintain balanced blood sugar levels.

3. Prepping in Advance: The Key to Success

Meal prepping is the practice of preparing ingredients or entire meals in advance to save time and reduce stress during the week. Prepping doesn't have to be overwhelming-start small by focusing on key ingredients that you can easily incorporate into different meals throughout the week.

How to get started:

Batch cook grains: Prepare a large batch of quinoa, brown rice, or farro at the beginning of the week. These can be used as a base for salads, grain bowls, or side dishes.

Prep your veggies: Wash and chop vegetables like carrots, bell peppers, zucchini, and leafy greens. Store them in airtight containers, so they're ready to be added to meals or enjoyed as snacks.

Cook proteins in bulk: Grill or bake a batch of lean proteins like chicken breast, turkey, or tofu. These can be used in wraps, salads, or grain bowls for quick and easy meals.

Make a big pot of soup: Soups like lentil, vegetable, or chicken and vegetable can be made in large quantities and stored in the fridge or freezer for easy lunches or dinners throughout the week.

Why it matters: Prepping ingredients ahead of time makes it easier to stick to your anti-inflammatory diet, even on busy days. It also ensures you always have healthy options at your fingertips, reducing the temptation to reach for processed or inflammatory foods.

4. Stay Flexible and Enjoy the Process

One of the most important aspects of meal planning is flexibility. Life can be unpredictable, and there will be days when you need to adjust your plan. That's okay! The key is to stay focused on making choices that nourish your body and support your anti-inflammatory goals.

How to stay flexible:Have backup meals or ingredients on hand for busy nights, like pre-cooked grains, canned beans, or frozen vegetables.

Don't stress if you have to change your plan—use what you have on hand to create simple, balanced meals.

Be creative and don't be afraid to experiment with new recipes, flavors, and ingredients.

Why it matters: Flexibility in meal planning helps reduce stress and keeps you motivated to stick to your anti-inflammatory diet in the long term. Remember, it's about progress, not perfection.

An anti-inflammatory diet is not a short-term fix but a long-term strategy for improving overall health, managing chronic diseases, and supporting the body's natural healing processes. By incorporating key anti-inflammatory foods into your daily meals, you can not only reduce inflammation but also enjoy a more vibrant, energized life. In this chapter, we'll explore some of the essential foods that form the foundation of an anti-inflammatory diet.

1. Leafy Greens: The Powerhouse of Nutrients

Leafy greens, such as kale, spinach, and Swiss chard, are rich in vitamins, minerals, and antioxidants. They provide high amounts of vitamin K, which is known for its anti-inflammatory properties. Additionally, these greens are loaded with fiber, which supports gut health, a crucial element in reducing inflammation throughout the body.

Why they matter: Leafy greens help lower markers of inflammation in the body, such as C-reactive protein (CRP). They also support cardiovascular health and aid in detoxifying the body.

How to incorporate them: Use them in salads, smoothies, soups, or stir-fries. The more greens you include in your daily diet, the better!

2. Fatty Fish: Omega-3 Superstars

Fatty fish like salmon, mackerel, sardines, and trout are some of the best sources of omega-3 fatty acids. These essential fats help reduce inflammation and are particularly beneficial for people with conditions like arthritis, cardiovascular disease, and autoimmune disorders. Omega-3s also improve brain health and can reduce the risk of depression.

Why they matter: Omega-3 fatty acids have been shown to significantly lower levels of inflammation in the body by reducing the production of inflammatory cytokines and enzymes.

How to incorporate them: Aim to include fatty fish in your diet at least twice a week. You can bake, grill, or broil fish, and pair it with anti-inflammatory vegetables for a well-rounded meal.

3. Berries: Antioxidant Powerhouses

Berries like blueberries, strawberries, and raspberries are packed with antioxidants called anthocyanins, which have strong anti-inflammatory effects. They also contain high levels of vitamin C, which helps the body combat oxidative stress – a key driver of inflammation.

Why they matter: Berries are known to reduce inflammatory markers and help improve insulin sensitivity, which is particularly beneficial for people with diabetes or those looking to manage their weight.

How to incorporate them: Add berries to your morning oatmeal, blend them into smoothies, or enjoy them as a snack throughout the day. Their natural sweetness also makes them a great alternative to sugary treats.

4. Turmeric: Nature's Golden Medicine

Turmeric is a potent anti-inflammatory spice, thanks to its active ingredient, curcumin. Studies have shown that curcumin can match the effectiveness of some anti-inflammatory drugs, without the side effects. This makes turmeric an excellent addition for those looking to reduce chronic inflammation, especially for conditions like arthritis and digestive disorders.

Why it matters: Curcumin helps block inflammatory molecules in the body, and regular consumption can significantly reduce pain and swelling associated with chronic inflammatory diseases.

How to incorporate it: Use turmeric in soups, curries, smoothies, or sprinkle it on roasted vegetables. To increase its absorption, pair turmeric with black pepper and a source of healthy fat, such as olive oil.

5. Nuts and Seeds: Tiny but Mighty

Nuts like almonds and walnuts, as well as seeds like flaxseeds and chia seeds, are rich in healthy fats, fiber, and magnesium – all of which help reduce inflammation. Walnuts, in particular, are high in alpha-linolenic acid (ALA), a type of omega-3 fatty acid that is beneficial for reducing inflammation in the cardiovascular system.

Why they matter: Nuts and seeds support heart health, reduce inflammatory markers, and help stabilize blood sugar levels, making them ideal for people with diabetes or metabolic issues.

How to incorporate them: Add a handful of nuts or seeds to salads, oatmeal, or yogurt. You can also use nut butters or flaxseed meal in smoothies for an extra nutrient boost.

6. Olive Oil: Liquid Gold for Heart Health

Extra virgin olive oil is a staple of the Mediterranean diet, known for its anti-inflammatory benefits. Olive oil is rich in monounsaturated fats and contains oleocanthal, a compound with similar effects to ibuprofen when it comes to reducing inflammation.

Why it matters: Olive oil helps protect the heart, reduces inflammation, and supports healthy cholesterol levels. It's an excellent fat source for cooking and salad dressings.

How to incorporate it: Use extra virgin olive oil for salad dressings, drizzle it over roasted vegetables, or sauté your food in it. Just make sure to choose high-quality, cold-pressed olive oil for the best benefits.

7. Whole Grains: Fuel for the Gut

Whole grains like quinoa, brown rice, and farro are excellent sources of fiber, which helps feed beneficial gut bacteria. A healthy gut is crucial for managing inflammation, as an imbalance in gut bacteria can trigger inflammatory responses in the body.

Why they matter: Whole grains have a lower glycemic index than refined grains, meaning they cause a slower, steadier release of sugar into the bloodstream. This helps prevent spikes in blood sugar that can lead to inflammation.

How to incorporate them: Swap out refined grains like white rice or pasta for whole grains in your meals. Try adding quinoa to salads, serving brown rice as a side dish, or incorporating oats into your breakfast.

8. Green Tea: A Soothing Anti-Inflammatory Drink

Green tea is rich in polyphenols, particularly epigallocatechin gallate (EGCG), which is known for its powerful anti-inflammatory effects. Drinking green tea regularly can help reduce inflammation, support weight loss, and improve brain function.

Why it matters: Green tea helps reduce inflammatory markers and is beneficial for cardiovascular health, as well as providing a gentle energy boost without the crash associated with coffee.

How to incorporate it: Enjoy a cup of green tea in the morning or afternoon. You can also use it as a base for smoothies or iced tea for a refreshing, anti-inflammatory drink.

Bringing it All Together

The beauty of an anti-inflammatory diet lies in the diversity and richness of the foods you can enjoy. By focusing on whole, nutrient-dense foods, you not only reduce inflammation but also nourish your body in a way that promotes long-term health. Whether you're dealing with a chronic condition like arthritis, or simply looking to boost your energy and well-being, incorporating these essential anti-inflammatory foods into your diet will help you thrive.

Adapting Recipes for People with Allergies

In today's world, food allergies are becoming more common, and this reality cannot be ignored, especially when you're focusing on healthy, anti-inflammatory eating. The good news is that many recipes, even those that are designed for a specific diet like the anti-inflammatory one, can be easily adapted for people with allergies. Whether you or your loved ones have allergies to common ingredients like dairy, gluten, nuts, or eggs, there are always healthy alternatives that allow you to enjoy the same delicious meals without compromising flavor or nutrition.

In this chapter, we'll walk through the common food allergies, how they relate to inflammation, and most importantly, how to modify recipes so that everyone at your table can enjoy the benefits of an anti-inflammatory diet safely and comfortably.

1. Understanding Common Food Allergies and Their Triggers

Before diving into how to adapt recipes, it's important to understand the most common food allergies that people may need to work around:

Dairy: Many people have lactose intolerance or are allergic to the proteins found in cow's milk. Dairy can also trigger inflammation in some individuals.

Gluten: Those with celiac disease or gluten intolerance experience digestive and immune responses when consuming gluten-containing grains like wheat, barley, and rye.

Eggs: Egg allergies are common, especially in children, and can cause digestive upset, skin issues, or respiratory problems.

Nuts and peanuts: Nut allergies can be severe and are often life-threatening. Even exposure to small amounts of peanuts or tree nuts can trigger a reaction.

Soy: While a healthy protein source for many, soy is another common allergen that can cause digestive and inflammatory issues for those sensitive to it.

Fish and shellfish: Seafood allergies are particularly common and can result in serious reactions. These allergens can be found in dishes that include fish or shellfish.

Why it matters: Understanding these common allergens is key to adapting recipes in a way that continues to reduce inflammation without triggering allergic reactions.

2. How to Swap Ingredients Without Sacrificing Flavor

One of the biggest challenges when adapting recipes for people with allergies is ensuring the final dish is still flavorful and nutritious. Luckily, there are many anti-inflammatory alternatives that can be used in place of allergenic ingredients.

For dairy: Replace cow's milk with non-dairy alternatives like almond milk, coconut milk, or oat milk. For yogurt, try coconut or almond-based versions. Nutritional yeast is a great substitute for cheese, adding a savory, "cheesy" flavor to dishes.

For gluten: Gluten-free grains like quinoa, brown rice, and millet are excellent substitutes for **Dairy-free options**: Ensure that calcium and vitamin D levels remain high by including fortified plant-based milks or leafy greens like kale and spinach.

wheat-based grains. For baking, you can use gluten-free flours made from almond, coconut, or rice.

For eggs: Use chia or flax seeds mixed with water to create an egg-like consistency for baking (1 tablespoon ground chia/flax seeds + 3 tablespoons water = 1 egg). Applesauce or mashed bananas can also work as egg replacements in some recipes.

For nuts: Sunflower seeds or pumpkin seeds can often stand in for nuts in salads, smoothies, or granola. For peanut butter, consider using sunflower seed butter or tahini.

For soy: If you're avoiding soy, you can use coconut aminos as a soy sauce substitute, and many plant-based meat alternatives are now soy-free.

For fish/shellfish: To replace seafood, consider using mushrooms or jackfruit for texture, or incorporate more plant-based proteins like beans or lentils to maintain protein content.

Why it matters: These substitutions not only keep meals safe for those with allergies but also maintain the anti-inflammatory benefits of the diet by using nutrient-dense alternatives.

3. Adjusting Recipes Without Losing Nutritional Value

When making swaps for allergens, it's important to consider the nutritional impact of those changes. For example, if you're eliminating nuts or seeds, you're losing a source of healthy fats and protein. If you're removing gluten, you may also lose some fiber from whole grains. Here's how you can make sure your meals remain balanced:

Gluten-free options: Boost fiber content by incorporating plenty of fresh vegetables and gluten-free whole grains like quinoa and buckwheat.

Egg-free options: If you're removing eggs, add extra plant-based protein sources such as beans, lentils, or hemp seeds.

Nut-free options: If nuts are off-limits, add healthy fats from avocados, olives, or flaxseed oil.

Why it matters: Swapping ingredients doesn't mean sacrificing nutrition. Being mindful of maintaining a balance of nutrients will keep your anti-inflammatory diet effective and fulfilling.

4. Customizing Meal Plans for People with Multiple Allergies

For those dealing with more than one food allergy, planning meals can seem like an overwhelming task. However, by sticking to whole, natural foods, it's easy to create a meal plan that avoids common allergens while still supporting an anti-inflammatory diet.

Here's an example of how to adapt a typical anti-inflammatory day of eating for someone avoiding dairy, gluten, and nuts:

Breakfast: Smoothie with unsweetened coconut milk, fresh berries, chia seeds, and spinach.

Lunch: Quinoa and kale salad with roasted sweet potatoes, avocado, and a lemon-tahini dressing.

Dinner: Baked salmon with roasted Brussels sprouts and quinoa.

Snack: Sliced cucumber with homemade hummus (made without tahini).

Why it matters: Customizing meal plans ensures that people with multiple allergies can still enjoy anti-inflammatory meals without feeling restricted or deprived.

5. Staying Safe in the Kitchen: Preventing Cross-Contamination

When preparing meals for someone with allergies, especially in a shared kitchen, it's crucial to take steps to prevent cross-contamination. Even trace amounts of allergens can trigger a reaction, so here are a few tips to keep your kitchen safe:

Separate cooking tools: Use separate cutting boards, knives, and cookware for allergen-free cooking to prevent cross-contact.

Store allergens separately: Keep foods that contain allergens in clearly labeled, separate containers to avoid accidental mixing.

Clean thoroughly: Make sure to clean all surfaces, cookware, and utensils thoroughly after cooking with allergenic ingredients.

Label leftovers: If storing leftovers, label them clearly so that family members know which meals are allergen-free.

Why it matters: Keeping your kitchen safe and organized ensures that meals remain truly allergy-friendly, protecting your loved ones from potential reactions.

6. Empowering Yourself with Knowledge and Flexibility

Adapting recipes for people with allergies may seem challenging at first, but with the right knowledge, it becomes second nature. Focus on what you can include in your meals rather than what you can't, and explore new ingredients and flavors along the way. There's no need to feel limited—many allergy-friendly alternatives are packed with nutrients and flavor, making them a perfect fit for an anti-inflammatory diet.

How to stay flexible:

Be open to experimenting with new ingredients.

Take inspiration from global cuisines that naturally avoid common allergens.

Don't hesitate to adjust recipes based on your or your family's specific needs.

Why it matters: When you empower yourself with knowledge and remain flexible in the kitchen, adapting an anti-inflammatory diet for allergies becomes an opportunity to discover new and delicious ways to nourish your body.

Stock Your Pantry Like a Pro

Your pantry is the foundation of your kitchen, and when it comes to following an anti-inflammatory diet, having the right ingredients at your fingertips is essential. With a well-stocked pantry, you'll be able to whip up healthy meals quickly and easily, without the stress of figuring out what to cook each day. In this chapter, we'll walk you through the must-have ingredients for an anti-inflammatory diet, how to organize your pantry for success, and tips for shopping smart while saving money.

1.Must-Have Ingredients

The key to an anti-inflammatory kitchen is having a variety of nutrient-rich staples on hand. These ingredients will help you build delicious, balanced meals that reduce inflammation and support your overall health.

1. **Healthy Fats**: Stock up on high-quality sources of healthy fats, which are essential for reducing inflammation. Some of the best options include:
   - Extra virgin olive oil
   - Avocados
   - Coconut oil
   - Nuts and seeds (almonds, chia seeds, flaxseeds, walnuts)
   - Nut butters (almond, cashew, peanut)
2. **Whole Grains**: Swap out refined grains for nutrient-dense whole grains that are packed with fiber and promote gut health. Make sure to have these on hand:
   - Quinoa
   - Brown rice
   - Oats
   - Buckwheat
   - Farro
   - Whole grain pasta
3. **Lean Proteins**: Anti-inflammatory proteins are essential for muscle repair and overall energy. Keep these pantry-friendly proteins stocked:
   - Canned beans (black beans, chickpeas, lentils)
   - Canned tuna or salmon
   - Dried lentils
   - Organic tofu or tempeh
4. **Herbs and Spices**: Herbs and spices are a key part of anti-inflammatory cooking. Not only do they add flavor, but many also have powerful anti-inflammatory properties. Make sure you have:
   - Turmeric
   - Ginger
   - Garlic powder
   - Cinnamon
   - Cayenne pepper
   - Oregano, thyme, and rosemary
5. **Fermented Foods**: Support gut health with fermented foods, which are rich in probiotics and help reduce inflammation. Keep these staples in your pantry or fridge:
   - Sauerkraut
   - Kimchi
   - Miso paste
   - Unsweetened yogurt
6. **Fresh and Frozen Produce**: While fresh fruits and vegetables are always great, frozen produce is a convenient option to ensure you have nutrient-dense ingredients available anytime. Stock your pantry and freezer with:
   - Frozen spinach, broccoli, and berries
   - Fresh garlic, onions, and sweet potatoes
   - Fresh leafy greens, bell peppers, and carrots

2.Organize for Success

A well-organized pantry is a game-changer when it comes to sticking to a healthy eating plan. When you can see and easily access everything you need, you'll be less likely to reach for unhealthy options or feel overwhelmed by meal prep. Here are a few tips to organize your pantry like a pro:

1. **Categorize by Food Group**: Keep similar ingredients together in clear categories. Group healthy fats like oils, nuts, and seeds together. Keep all grains in one section and beans or proteins in another. This makes meal prep faster and helps you see what you have on hand.

2. **Use Clear Containers**: Transfer bulk items like grains, nuts, and seeds into clear, airtight containers. This not only keeps them fresh but also allows you to see exactly how much you have. Bonus: it looks great and makes your pantry feel organized.

3. **Label Everything**: Don't underestimate the power of labeling. Use simple labels on jars or containers to ensure you can quickly find what you're looking for. This will save you time when cooking and make restocking easier.

4. **Rotate Ingredients**: Always place newer items behind older ones, so you use up ingredients before they expire. This is especially important for oils, nuts, and grains, which can lose their freshness over time.

5. **Keep Your Pantry Tidy**: Dedicate a few minutes each week to tidy up your pantry, toss expired products, and restock key items. A clean and organized pantry will motivate you to cook more and enjoy the process.

3.Shop Smart and Save

Stocking your pantry for an anti-inflammatory diet doesn't have to break the bank. With a few smart shopping strategies, you can build a well-stocked kitchen while saving money. Here's how:

1. **Buy in Bulk**: Buying staple ingredients like grains, nuts, seeds, and beans in bulk can save you a significant amount of money. Check if your local grocery store offers bulk bins, or shop online for larger quantities at lower prices.

2. **Shop Seasonal**: Seasonal produce is often cheaper and fresher. Build your meals around what's in season to save money and enjoy the best-tasting ingredients. For example, stock up on berries in summer or root vegetables like sweet potatoes in winter.

3. **Frozen is Your Friend**: Don't hesitate to buy frozen fruits and vegetables. They are usually flash-frozen at their peak freshness, making them just as nutritious as fresh produce—and often more affordable. Keep frozen spinach, berries, and broccoli in your freezer for easy access.

4. **Use Store Brands**: Many store-brand versions of whole grains, beans, and frozen vegetables are just as high-quality as name brands, but come at a lower cost. Don't be afraid to opt for store brands when stocking up on pantry essentials.

5. **Shop Sales and Use Coupons**: Keep an eye on weekly sales and take advantage of discounts on items you regularly use. Many grocery stores offer digital coupons or discounts through their apps, so be sure to check before heading to the store.

6. **Meal Plan Before Shopping**: Plan your meals for the week before heading to the store. By knowing exactly what ingredients you need, you can avoid impulse purchases and reduce food waste. Plus, it makes shopping faster and more efficient.

By stocking your pantry with the right ingredients, organizing it for success, and shopping smart, you'll set yourself up for success on your anti-inflammatory journey. With these tools and tips, preparing healthy, delicious meals will become second nature, allowing you to enjoy the process and reap the benefits of a well-balanced, anti-inflammatory diet.

CHAPTER 2: JUMP INTO YOUR 30-DAY PLAN

This structured 30-day plan is designed to ease you into an anti-inflammatory lifestyle, week by week. Each week, you'll focus on different aspects of the diet, ensuring that the changes you make are manageable, enjoyable, and effective. Follow this plan to gradually reduce inflammation, boost energy, and improve overall health.

Week 1: Transition with Ease

Goal: Begin to eliminate the most common inflammatory foods and replace them with whole, nutrient-dense options.

Day 1-3:

- **Remove Processed Foods**: Begin by cutting out highly processed snacks, sugary drinks, and refined carbohydrates.
- **Start Adding Whole Foods**: Replace them with whole grains (quinoa, brown rice), lean proteins (chicken, turkey, tofu), and a variety of vegetables (leafy greens, broccoli, peppers).

Day 4-7:

- **Focus on Hydration**: Drink at least 8 glasses of water per day, and switch from sugary drinks to herbal teas or water with lemon.
- **Snack Smart**: Replace unhealthy snacks with nuts, seeds, fruits, or vegetable sticks with hummus.
- **Start Your Day with Protein**: Incorporate a high-protein breakfast such as eggs, a smoothie with protein powder, or Greek yogurt with berries.

Week 2: Add Flavor and Nutrition

Goal: Add anti-inflammatory herbs and spices to your meals and increase your intake of colorful fruits and vegetables.

Day 8-10:

- **Introduce Anti-Inflammatory Spices**: Add turmeric, ginger, and garlic to your meals. For example, add turmeric to a smoothie, ginger to a stir-fry, and garlic to roasted vegetables.
- **Increase Your Fiber Intake**: Start including fiber-rich foods like oats, lentils, beans, and leafy greens in your meals.

Day 11-14:

- **Boost Your Color Intake**: Make sure your plate is colorful with a variety of fruits and vegetables. Aim to include at least three different colors in each meal (e.g., red peppers, orange sweet potatoes, and green spinach).
- **Experiment with Flavors**: Try new herbs such as rosemary, thyme, and cilantro to season your dishes.

Week 3: Power Up with Superfoods

Goal: Incorporate nutrient-dense superfoods into your diet to supercharge your body's healing process.

Day 15-17:

- **Add Omega-3s**: Incorporate more foods rich in omega-3 fatty acids like salmon, chia seeds, flaxseeds, and walnuts. Aim to have fatty fish at least twice this week.
- **Focus on Antioxidants**: Add antioxidant-rich foods like blueberries, spinach, and dark chocolate (70% cacao or higher).

Day 18-21:

- **Include Fermented Foods**: Start adding fermented foods like sauerkraut, kimchi, or yogurt to support gut health.
- **Add Seeds and Nuts**: Sprinkle chia seeds or flaxseeds onto salads, smoothies, or oatmeal to increase fiber and omega-3 intake.

Week 4: Create Lasting Habits

Goal: Solidify your anti-inflammatory eating habits and focus on meal planning and prepping for long-term success.

Day 22-24:

- **Plan and Prep**: Begin creating a meal plan for the upcoming week and batch cook some meals on the weekend. Prep grains, roast vegetables, and portion out snacks to save time during busy days.
- **Keep Your Pantry Stocked**: Make sure you have all the essentials for anti-inflammatory cooking: olive oil, fresh herbs, spices, nuts, seeds, and whole grains.

Day 25-30:

- **Maintain Variety**: Experiment with new recipes and ingredients to keep things exciting and avoid food boredom. Continue exploring new superfoods and flavor combinations.
- **Consistency Over Perfection**: Focus on consistency rather than perfection. Don't worry if you slip up, just get back on track with your next meal.

Tips for Success:

- **Meal Prep**: Batch cook on Sundays to ensure you have healthy meals ready for the week.
- **Keep it Simple**: Don't overcomplicate your meals. Simple, whole foods with basic seasonings can still be delicious and effective in reducing inflammation.
- **Listen to Your Body**: Pay attention to how you feel after eating certain foods. You may discover which specific ingredients help you feel your best.

By following this plan, you'll not only reduce inflammation but also develop lasting habits that will improve your overall health and well-being. This structured approach makes it easy to transition into a healthier, anti-inflammatory lifestyle while enjoying delicious and nutritious meals every step of the way.

30-DAY PLAN

Day	Breakfast (600 kcal)	Lunch (600 kcal)	Snack (400 kcal)	Dinner (400 kcal)
1	Matcha Green Power Smoothie - p.23	Blueberry Almond Arugula Salad with Goat Cheese - p.36	Peanut Butter Banana Rice Cakes - p.62	Miso Glazed Salmon with Bok Choy - p.49
2	Golden Turmeric Cashew Oatmeal - p.27	Zesty Lime Barley Bowl with Grilled Peppers - p.39	Roasted Beet Chips with Sea Salt - p.62	Sweet Potato & Black Bean Tacos with Avocado - p.53
3	Roasted Asparagus & Goat Cheese Omelette - p.29	Grilled Chicken & Avocado Romaine Crunch Salad - p.37	Zucchini Muffins with Walnuts and Cinnamon - p.63	Garlic Butter Tilapia with Steamed Broccoli - p.50
4	Cranberry Orange Zest Oatmeal - p.26	Honey Dijon Chicken & Apple Salad - p.37	Chia Seed Pudding with Mango - p.63	Coconut Lime Shrimp with Cilantro Rice - p.51
5	Papaya Ginger Digestive Smoothie - p.24	Chili-Lime Shrimp & Avocado Lettuce Wrap - p.42	Almond Butter and Berry Oat Bars - p.64	Spicy Beef Stir Fry with Zucchini Noodles - p.59
6	Berry Bliss Oats with Hemp Seeds - p.26	Smoked Salmon & Avocado Arugula Salad - p.38	Pumpkin Seed Protein Bars with Cacao - p.64	Teriyaki Salmon Stir Fry with Bok Choy - p.60
7	Broccoli Cheddar Breakfast Bake - p.29	Sweet Potato & Kale Freekeh Bowl - p.39	Spicy Black Bean Dip with Cilantro and Lime - p.66	Paprika Chicken with Roasted Broccoli and Carrots - p.56
8	Zucchini Noodles & Pesto Eggs - p.30	Curried Chickpea & Carrot Wrap - p.44	Cucumber & Dill Yogurt Spread - p.66	Sheet Pan Cod with Lemon and Dill Potatoes - p.57
9	Apple Cinnamon Protein Smoothie - p.23	Spicy Shrimp & Mango Spinach Salad - p.38	Roasted Red Peppers with Garlic and Thyme - p.68	Balsamic Glazed Mushroom & Farro Stir Fry - p.54
10	Pear & Pumpkin Seed Oatmeal - p.27	Lemon Garlic Bulgur Bowl with Zucchini - p.40	Caramelized Beets with Balsamic Vinegar - p.70	Coconut Ginger Tofu Stir Fry with Kale - p.61
11	Spinach Avocado Egg Wrap - p.32	Grilled Veggie & Hummus Wrap - p.44	Sweet Potato & Roasted Garlic Hummus - p.67	Spiced Salmon with Cucumber Dill Salad - p.49
12	Blueberry Spinach Antioxidant Smoothie - p.25	Avocado & Sriracha Millet Bowl - p.41	Zucchini Basil Pesto with Almonds - p.65	One-Pan Spicy Tempeh with Bell Peppers - p.58
13	Cacao Hazelnut Dream Oatmeal - p.28	Roasted Sweet Potato & Black Bean Power Salad - p.36	Pumpkin and Carrot Tahini Dip with Cumin - p.65	Miso Veggie Stir Fry with Cashews - p.61
14	Eggplant Tomato Shakshuka Delight - p.31	Grilled Chicken & Hummus Lettuce Wrap - p.43	Cucumber & Dill Yogurt Spread - p.66	Crispy Tofu with Roasted Cauliflower and Carrots - p.58
15	Ginger Turmeric Pancakes - p.33	Toasted Buckwheat Bowl with Mushrooms & Spinach - p.40	Roasted Beet Chips with Sea Salt - p.62	Thyme-Roasted Chicken with Carrots and Parsnips - p.52

Day	Breakfast (600 kcal)	Lunch (600 kcal)	Snack (400 kcal)	Dinner (400 kcal)
16	Avocado Kiwi Gut Health Smoothie - p.24	Sweet Potato & Kale Freekeh Bowl - p.39	Almond Butter and Berry Oat Bars - p.64	Balsamic Glazed Mushroom & Farro Stir Fry - p.54
17	Bell Pepper & Turkey Bacon Egg Muffins - p.32	Zucchini & Goat Cheese Lettuce Wrap - p.43	Chia Seed Pudding with Mango - p.63	Garlic Butter Tilapia with Steamed Broccoli - p.50
18	Golden Cinnamon Spice Pancakes - p.35	Crispy Chickpea & Barley Buddha Bowl - p.41	Peanut Butter Banana Rice Cakes - p.62	Turmeric-Crusted Cod with Quinoa - p.51
19	Blueberry Spinach Antioxidant Smoothie - p.25	Roasted Sweet Potato & Black Bean Power Salad - p.36	Roasted Red Peppers with Garlic and Thyme - p.68	Coconut Lime Shrimp with Cilantro Rice - p.51
20	Coconut Quinoa Protein Pancakes - p.34	Grilled Chicken & Avocado Romaine Crunch Salad - p.37	Zucchini Muffins with Walnuts and Cinnamon - p.63	Paprika Chicken with Roasted Broccoli and Carrots - p.56
21	Matcha Green Tea Pancakes with Berries - p.33	Smoked Salmon & Avocado Arugula Salad - p.38	Pumpkin Seed Protein Bars with Cacao - p.64	Spicy Beef Stir Fry with Zucchini Noodles - p.59
22	Zesty Kale & Tomato Scramble - p.30	Grilled Chicken & Hummus Lettuce Wrap - p.43	Roasted Beet Chips with Sea Salt - p.62	Butternut Squash and Black Bean Enchiladas - p.55
23	Egg-Stuffed Bell Pepper Rings - p.31	Chili-Lime Shrimp & Avocado Lettuce Wrap - p.42	Cucumber & Dill Yogurt Spread - p.66	Sweet Potato & Black Bean Tacos with Avocado - p.53
24	Chocolate Hazelnut Superfood Pancakes - p.35	Lemon Garlic Bulgur Bowl with Zucchini - p.40	Spicy Black Bean Dip with Cilantro and Lime - p.66	Coconut Curry Lentil Stew with Cauliflower - p.53
25	Golden Turmeric Cashew Oatmeal - p.27	Blueberry Almond Arugula Salad with Goat Cheese - p.36	Chia Seed Pudding with Mango - p.63	Crispy Tofu with Ginger Sesame Spinach - p.55
26	Pineapple Kale Cleansing Smoothie - p.25	Avocado & Sriracha Millet Bowl - p.41	Zucchini Muffins with Walnuts and Cinnamon - p.63	Turmeric-Roasted Vegetables with Chicken Thighs - p.56
27	Avocado Kiwi Gut Health Smoothie - p.24	Honey Dijon Chicken & Apple Salad - p.37	Roasted Beet Chips with Sea Salt - p.62	Miso Glazed Salmon with Bok Choy - p.49
28	Cacao Hazelnut Dream Oatmeal - p.28	Smoked Salmon & Avocado Arugula Salad - p.38	Almond Butter and Berry Oat Bars - p.64	Garlic Butter Tilapia with Steamed Broccoli - p.50
29	Berry Bliss Oats with Hemp Seeds - p.26	Crispy Chickpea & Barley Buddha Bowl - p.41	Peanut Butter Banana Rice Cakes - p.62	Coconut Ginger Tofu Stir Fry with Kale - p.61
30	Papaya Ginger Digestive Smoothie - p.24	Curried Chickpea & Carrot Wrap - p.44	Cucumber & Dill Yogurt Spread - p.66	One-Pan Garlic Shrimp with Zucchini Noodles - p.57

CHAPTER 3: COOK FAST AND ENJOY

Fuel Your Day with Power Breakfast:Boost with Smoothies

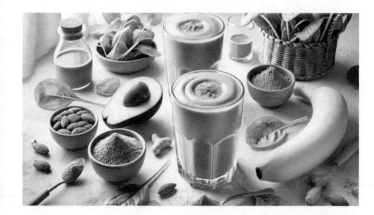

Matcha Green Power Smoothie

Prep: 5 minutes **Cook: N/A** **Serves: 2**

Ingredients:

- 2 cups (480 ml) unsweetened almond milk
- 1 tbsp (6g) matcha powder
- 1 frozen banana (120g)
- 1/2 avocado (75g)
- 1/2 cup (75g) spinach
- 1 tbsp (15 ml) flaxseed oil (optional for omega-3)
- 1/2 tsp (2g) ground turmeric
- 1 tbsp (15 ml) lemon juice
- 1 tsp (5g) honey or agave syrup (optional)

Instructions:

1. **Blend ingredients**: Combine almond milk, matcha powder, banana, avocado, spinach, flaxseed oil, turmeric, lemon juice, and honey in a blender.
2. **Blend until smooth**: Blend for about 1 minute until creamy.
3. **Serve**: Pour into two glasses and serve immediately.

Nutritional Facts (Per Serving):
Calories: 210 | Carbs: 30g | Protein: 4g | Fat: 9g | Sugar: 12g

Variations and Tips

For diabetics: Replace the banana with 1/4 avocado to reduce the sugar content.
For allergies: Omit flaxseed oil or replace it with 1 tbsp (15 ml) of olive oil.
Flavor tip: Add 5–6 mint leaves or 1/2 tsp grated ginger for freshness.

Apple Cinnamon Protein Smoothie

Prep: 5 minutes **Cook: N/A** **Serves: 2**

Ingredients:

- 1 large apple (180g), chopped
- 1/2 frozen banana (60g)
- 1/2 cup (120 ml) unsweetened oat milk
- 1/2 tsp (2g) ground cinnamon
- 1 tbsp (15 ml) chia seeds
- 1 tbsp (15 ml) almond butter
- 1/2 tsp (2g) vanilla extract
- 1/2 cup (120 ml) water or ice

Instructions:

1. **Blend ingredients**: Combine apple, banana, oat milk, cinnamon, ginger, chia seeds, almond butter, vanilla, and water (or ice) in a blender.
2. **Blend until smooth**: Blend for about 1 minute until creamy.
3. **Serve**: Pour into two glasses and serve immediately.

Nutritional Facts (Per Serving):
Calories: 250 | Carbs: 38g | Protein:6g | Fat:10g | Sugar: 18g

Variations and Tips

For diabetics: Reduce apple to 1/2 (90g) and replace the banana with 1/4 avocado.
For allergies: Replace almond butter with 1 tbsp (15 ml) sunflower seed butter.
Flavor tip: Add 1/4 tsp nutmeg for a stronger fall flavor.

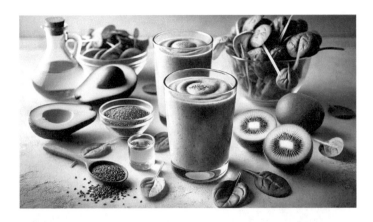

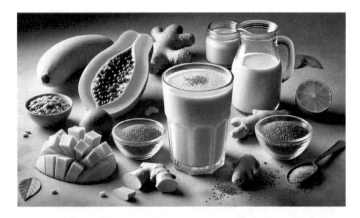

Avocado Kiwi Gut Health Smoothie

| Prep: 5 minutes | Cook: N/A | Serves: 2 |

Ingredients:

- 1 ripe avocado (150g)
- 2 ripe kiwis (140g), peeled
- 1/2 frozen banana (60g)
- 1 cup (240 ml) unsweetened coconut water
- 1 tbsp (15 ml) flaxseed oil (for omega-3 boost)
- 1/2 cup (75g) spinach
- 1/2 tsp (2g) ground ginger (anti-inflammatory boost)
- 1 tbsp (15 ml) lemon juice

Instructions:

1. **Blend ingredients**: Combine avocado, kiwis, banana, coconut water, flaxseed oil, spinach, ground ginger, and lemon juice in a blender.
2. **Blend until smooth**: Blend for 1 minute or until smooth and creamy.
3. **Serve**: Pour into two glasses and serve immediately

Nutritional Facts (Per Serving):
Calories: 250 | Carbs: 23g | Protein: 3g | Fat: 18g | Sugar: 12g

Variations and Tips

For diabetics: Replace the banana with 1/4 extra avocado to lower sugar content.
For allergies: Omit flaxseed oil or replace it with 1 tbsp (15 ml) olive oil.
Flavor tip: Add a few mint leaves or a pinch of turmeric for added freshness and anti-inflammatory benefits.

Papaya Ginger Digestive Smoothie

| Prep: 5 minutes | Cook: N/A | Serves: 2 |

Ingredients:

- 1 cup (140g) papaya, chopped
- 1/2 frozen banana (60g)
- 1/2 cup (120 ml) unsweetened almond milk
- 1/2 cup (120 ml) water or ice
- 1 tbsp (15 ml) chia seeds (for fiber and omega-3)
- 1/2 tsp (2g) ground ginger
- 1 tsp (5 ml) honey or agave syrup (optional)
- 1 tbsp (15 ml) fresh lime juice

Instructions:

1. **Blend ingredients**: Combine papaya, banana, almond milk, water (or ice), chia seeds, ground ginger, honey, and lime juice in a blender.
2. **Blend until smooth**: Blend for 1 minute or until smooth and creamy.
3. **Serve**: Pour into two glasses and serve immediately.

Nutritional Facts (Per Serving):
Calories: 210 | Carbs: 32g | Protein: 4g | Fat: 8g |Sugar: 18g

Variations and Tips

For diabetics: Reduce the banana to 1/4 (30g) and replace with extra papaya.
For those with allergies: Use coconut milk instead of almond milk.
Flavor tip: Add a dash of cinnamon or turmeric for additional digestive and anti-inflammatory benefits.

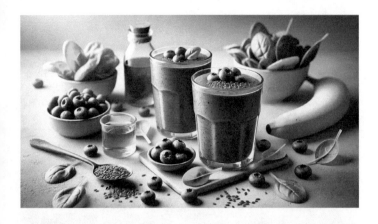

Blueberry Spinach Antioxidant Smoothie

Prep: 5 minutes   **Cook: N/A**   **Serves: 2**

Ingredients:

- 1 cup (150g) fresh or frozen blueberries
- 1/2 frozen banana (60g)
- 1 cup (240 ml) unsweetened almond milk
- 1/2 cup (75g) spinach
- 1 tbsp (15 ml) flaxseed oil (for omega-3 boost)
- 1 tbsp (15 ml) lemon juice
- 1/2 tsp (2g) ground turmeric (anti-inflammatory boost)
- 1 tbsp (15 ml) chia seeds (optional for added fiber)

Instructions:

1. **Blend ingredients**: Combine blueberries, banana, almond milk, spinach, flaxseed oil, lemon juice, turmeric, and chia seeds in a blender.
2. **Blend until smooth**: Blend for 1 minute or until smooth and creamy.
3. **Serve**: Pour into two glasses and serve immediatel

Nutritional Facts (Per Serving):
Calories: 220 | Carbs: 28g | Protein: 4g | Fat: 11g | Sugar: 15g

Variations and Tips

For diabetics: Reduce the banana to 1/4 (30g) to lower sugar content.
For allergies: Replace flaxseed oil with 1 tbsp (15 ml) olive oil.
Flavor tip: Add a pinch of cinnamon or ginger for a flavor kick and additional anti-inflammatory benefits.

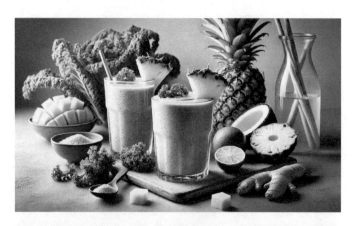

Pineapple Kale Cleansing Smoothie

Prep: 5 minutes   **Cook: N/A**   **Serves: 2**

Ingredients:

- 1 cup (160g) fresh or frozen pineapple
- 1/2 cup (75g) kale, chopped
- 1/2 frozen banana (60g)
- 1 cup (240 ml) coconut water
- 1 tbsp (15 ml) flaxseed oil (for omega-3)
- 1/2 tbsp (7 ml) fresh lime juice
- 1/2 tsp (2g) ground ginger

Instructions:

1. **Blend ingredients**: Combine pineapple, kale, banana, coconut water, flaxseed oil, lime juice, and ginger in a blender.
2. **Blend until smooth**: Blend for about 1 minute until creamy and smooth.
3. **Serve**: Pour into two glasses and enjoy immediately.

Nutritional Facts (Per Serving):
Calories: 230 | Carbs: 32g | Protein: 3g | Fat: 9g | Sugar: 20g

Variations and Tips

For diabetics: Reduce pineapple to 1/2 cup (80g) and replace banana with 1/4 avocado to lower sugar.
For allergies: Use olive oil instead of flaxseed oil.
Flavor tip: Add a few mint leaves or a pinch of cayenne pepper for an extra kick.

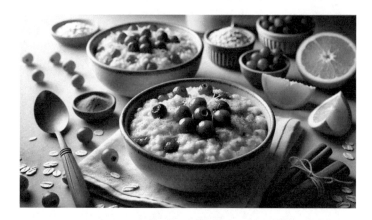

Cranberry Orange Zest Oatmeal

Prep: 5 minutes   Cook: 10 minutes   Serves: 2

Ingredients:

- 1 cup (90g) rolled oats
- 2 cups (480 ml) unsweetened almond milk
- 1/2 cup (50g) fresh or frozen cranberries
- 1 tbsp (15 ml) maple syrup (optional)
- 1 tsp (5g) orange zest
- 1/2 tsp (2g) ground cinnamon (anti-inflammatory boost)
- 1 tbsp (15 ml) chia seeds (optional for added fiber and omega-3)

Instructions:

1. **Cook oats**: In a small pot, combine the oats, almond milk, and cranberries. Bring to a simmer over medium heat.
2. **Simmer**: Cook for 8-10 minutes, stirring occasionally until the oats are creamy and the cranberries have softened.
3. **Add flavor**: Stir in the maple syrup, orange zest, cinnamon, and chia seeds.
4. **Serve**: Divide between two bowls and serve warm.

Nutritional Facts (Per Serving):
Calories: 230 | Carbs: 38g | Protein: 6g | Fat: 7g | Sugar: 12g

Variations and Tips

For diabetics: Reduce or omit maple syrup and replace cranberries with blueberries for lower sugar content.
For allergies: Replace almond milk with oat or coconut milk.
Flavor tip: Add a pinch of nutmeg or ginger for an extra spice boost

Berry Bliss Oats with Hemp Seeds

Prep: 5 minutes   Cook: 10 minutes   Serves: 2

Ingredients:

- 1 cup (90g) rolled oats
- 2 cups (480 ml) unsweetened oat milk
- 1/2 cup (75g) mixed berries (fresh or frozen)
- 1 tbsp (15 ml) hemp seeds
- 1 tbsp (15 ml) maple syrup (optional)
- 1/2 tsp (2g) ground turmeric (anti-inflammatory boost)
- 1 tbsp (15 ml) ground flaxseed (optional for added fiber)

Instructions:

1. **Cook oats**: Combine oats and oat milk in a small pot. Bring to a simmer over medium heat.
2. **Simmer**: Stir occasionally and cook for 8-10 minutes until the oats are creamy and fully cooked.
3. **Add flavor**: Stir in the berries, hemp seeds, maple syrup, turmeric, and ground flaxseed.
4. **Serve**: Divide the oatmeal between two bowls and top with extra berries if desired

Nutritional Facts (Per Serving):
Calories: 240 | Carbs: 40g | Protein: 7g | Fat: 8g |Sugar: 10g

Variations and Tips

For diabetics: Use unsweetened berries and omit maple syrup.
For allergies: Replace oat milk with almond or coconut milk.
Flavor tip: Add a few crushed walnuts or almonds for a crunchy texture.

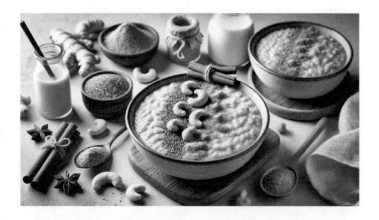

Golden Turmeric Cashew Oatmeal

Prep: 5 minutes   **Cook: 10 minutes**   **Serves: 2**

Ingredients:

- 1 cup (90g) rolled oats
- 2 cups (480 ml) unsweetened cashew milk
- 1 tbsp (15 ml) maple syrup (optional)
- 1/2 tsp (2g) ground turmeric (anti-inflammatory boost)
- 1/4 tsp (1g) ground ginger
- 1/2 tsp (2g) cinnamon
- 2 tbsp (30g) chopped cashews
- 1 tbsp (15 ml) chia seeds (optional for added fiber and omega-3)

Instructions:

1. **Cook oats**: Combine oats and cashew milk in a small pot. Bring to a simmer over medium heat.
2. **Simmer**: Stir occasionally and cook for 8-10 minutes until the oats are creamy and fully cooked.
3. **Add flavor**: Stir in the maple syrup, turmeric, ginger, cinnamon, chopped cashews, and chia seeds.
4. **Serve**: Divide into two bowls and serve warm

Nutritional Facts (Per Serving):
Calories: 240 | Carbs: 35g | Protein: 6g | Fat: 9g | Sugar: 10g

Variations and Tips

For diabetics: Omit the maple syrup and replace with a few drops of stevia or a sugar-free alternative.
For allergies: Replace cashew milk with almond or coconut milk.
Flavor tip: Top with extra cinnamon or add a pinch of black pepper to enhance turmeric absorption

Pear & Pumpkin Seed Oatmeal

Prep: 5 minutes   **Cook: 10 minutes**   **Serves: 2**

Ingredients:

- 1 cup (90g) rolled oats
- 2 cups (480 ml) unsweetened almond milk
- 1 ripe pear (150g), chopped
- 1 tbsp (15 ml) maple syrup (optional)
- 2 tbsp (30g) pumpkin seeds
- 1/2 tsp (2g) ground cinnamon
- 1 tbsp (15 ml) ground flaxseed (optional for added fiber)

Instructions:

1. **Cook oats**: Combine oats and almond milk in a small pot. Bring to a simmer over medium heat.
2. **Simmer**: Stir occasionally and cook for 8-10 minutes until the oats are creamy.
3. **Add flavor**: Stir in the chopped pear, maple syrup, pumpkin seeds, cinnamon, and flaxseed.
4. **Serve**: Divide into two bowls and enjoy

Nutritional Facts (Per Serving):
Calories: 250 | Carbs: 40g | Protein: 7g | Fat: 9g | Sugar: 14g

Variations and Tips

For diabetics: Use half of the pear and omit maple syrup to reduce sugar content.
For allergies: Replace almond milk with oat or coconut milk.
Flavor tip: Add a sprinkle of nutmeg or cardamom for a more complex flavor profile

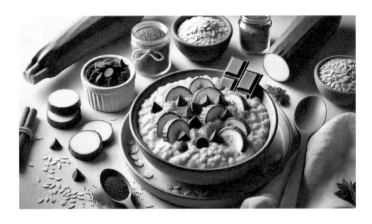

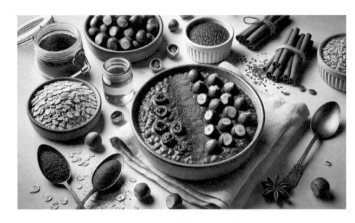

Zucchini Chocolate Chip Protein Oats

Prep: 5 minutes   Cook: 10 minutes   Serves: 2

Ingredients:

- 1 cup (90g) rolled oats
- 2 cups (480 ml) unsweetened almond milk
- 1/2 medium zucchini (100g), grated
- 2 tbsp (30g) dark chocolate chips (at least 70% cacao)
- 1 tbsp (15g) chia seeds (for added fiber and omega-3)
- 1 tbsp (15 ml) maple syrup (optional)
- 1/2 tsp (2g) ground cinnamon

Instructions:

1. **Cook oats**: In a small pot, combine the oats, almond milk, and grated zucchini. Bring to a simmer over medium heat.
2. **Simmer**: Stir occasionally and cook for 8-10 minutes until the oats are creamy.
3. **Add flavor**: Stir in the chocolate chips, chia seeds, maple syrup, and cinnamon.
4. **Serve**: Divide into two bowls and serve warm

Nutritional Facts (Per Serving):
Calories: 250 | Carbs: 38g | Protein: 7g | Fat: 9g |Sugar: 10g

Variations and Tips

For diabetics: Omit the maple syrup and use unsweetened dark chocolate to reduce sugar.
For allergies: Replace almond milk with oat or coconut milk.
Flavor tip: Add a pinch of nutmeg or vanilla extract for extra depth of flavor

Cacao Hazelnut Dream Oatmeal

Prep: 5 minutes   Cook: 10 minutes   Serves: 2

Ingredients:

- 1 cup (90g) rolled oats
- 2 cups (480 ml) unsweetened oat milk
- 1 tbsp (15g) cacao powder
- 2 tbsp (30g) chopped hazelnuts
- 1 tbsp (15 ml) maple syrup (optional)
- 1/2 tsp (2g) ground cinnamon
- 1 tbsp (15 ml) flaxseed oil (optional for omega-3 boost)

Instructions:

1. **Cook oats**: Combine the oats and oat milk in a small pot. Bring to a simmer over medium heat.
2. **Simmer**: Cook for 8-10 minutes, stirring occasionally, until creamy.
3. **Add flavor**: Stir in cacao powder, hazelnuts, maple syrup, cinnamon, and flaxseed oil.
4. **Serve**: Divide into two bowls and enjoy

Nutritional Facts (Per Serving):
Calories: 270 | Carbs: 40g | Protein:8g | Fat:11g | Sugar: 12g

Variations and Tips

For diabetics: Reduce or omit maple syrup and opt for a sugar-free sweetener.
For allergies: Use almond milk or coconut milk instead of oat milk.
Flavor tip: Add a pinch of cardamom or vanilla extract to enhance the cacao and nut flavors.

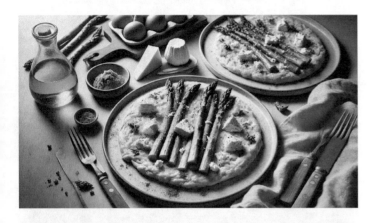

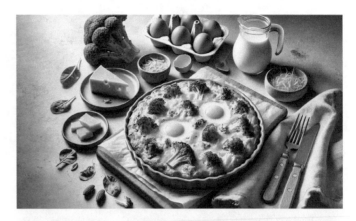

Roasted Asparagus & Goat Cheese Omelette

Prep: 5 minutes   **Cook: 10 minutes**   **Serves: 2**

Ingredients:

- 4 large eggs
- 1/2 cup (60g) asparagus, trimmed and chopped
- 2 tbsp (30g) goat cheese, crumbled
- 1 tbsp (15 ml) olive oil
- 1/4 tsp (1g) ground turmeric (anti-inflammatory boost)
- Salt and pepper to taste

Instructions:

1. **Roast asparagus**: Preheat the oven to 400°F (200°C). Toss the chopped asparagus with olive oil, salt, and pepper, then roast on a baking sheet for 10-12 minutes until tender.
2. **Whisk eggs**: In a bowl, whisk the eggs with turmeric, salt, and pepper.
3. **Cook omelette**: Heat a non-stick pan over medium heat. Pour in the eggs and cook for 2-3 minutes, gently stirring until the eggs begin to set.
4. **Add fillings**: Add roasted asparagus and crumbled goat cheese to one half of the omelette. Fold the omelette in half and cook for another 1-2 minutes until the cheese is slightly melted.
5. **Serve**: Divide the omelette into two portions and serve warm.

Nutritional Facts (Per Serving):
Calories: 220 | Carbs: 4g | Protein: 15g | Fat: 17g | Sugar: 2g

Variations and Tips

For vegetarians: This recipe is already vegetarian-friendly.
For allergies: Replace goat cheese with a dairy-free cheese alternative.
Flavor tip: Sprinkle fresh herbs like dill or parsley for an extra fresh kick.

Broccoli Cheddar Breakfast Bake

Prep: 5 minutes   **Cook: 25 minutes**   **Serves: 2**

Ingredients:

- 1 cup (90g) broccoli florets, chopped
- 4 large eggs
- 1/3 cup (40g) shredded cheddar cheese
- 1/4 cup (60 ml) unsweetened almond milk
- 1 tbsp (15 ml) olive oil
- 1/4 tsp (1g) ground black pepper
- Salt to taste

Instructions:

1. **Preheat oven**: Preheat the oven to 375°F (190°C) and lightly grease a small baking dish with olive oil.
2. **Cook broccoli**: In a pan over medium heat, sauté the broccoli with olive oil for 3-4 minutes until softened.
3. **Whisk eggs**: In a bowl, whisk together the eggs, almond milk, salt, and pepper.
4. **Assemble the bake**: Add the sautéed broccoli to the baking dish and pour the egg mixture over it. Sprinkle cheddar cheese on top.
5. **Bake**: Bake for 20-25 minutes until the eggs are set and the cheese is golden.
6. **Serve**: Cut the bake into two portions and serve warm.

Nutritional Facts (Per Serving):
Calories: 240 | Carbs: 40g | Protein: 7g | Fat: 8g | Sugar: 10g

Variations and Tips

For diabetics: Use unsweetened berries and omit maple syrup.
For allergies: Replace oat milk with almond or coconut milk.
Flavor tip: Add a few crushed walnuts or almonds for a crunchy texture.

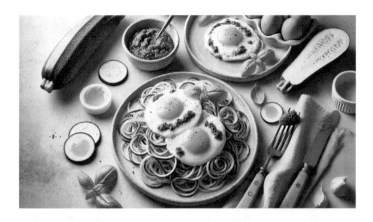

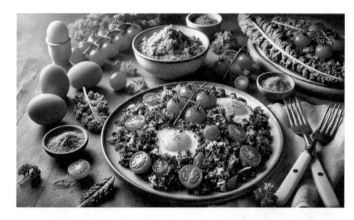

Zucchini Noodles & Pesto Eggs

Prep: 10 minutes   Cook: 10 minutes   Serves: 2

Ingredients:

- 2 medium zucchini (300g), spiralized
- 4 large eggs
- 2 tbsp (30g) pesto (homemade or store-bought)
- 1 tbsp (15 ml) olive oil
- 1/4 tsp (1g) ground black pepper
- Salt to taste
- Fresh basil for garnish (optional)

Instructions:

1. **Cook zucchini noodles**: Heat olive oil in a large pan over medium heat. Add spiralized zucchini noodles and cook for 2-3 minutes until softened. Season with salt and pepper.
2. **Cook eggs**: In a separate pan, heat a small amount of oil over medium heat. Crack the eggs and cook them to your preferred doneness (sunny side up or scrambled).
3. **Combine**: Plate the zucchini noodles and top with the cooked eggs. Drizzle with pesto.
4. **Serve**: Garnish with fresh basil if desired and serve warm.

Nutritional Facts (Per Serving):
Calories: 220 | Carbs: 6g | Protein: 14g | Fat: 17g |Sugar: 3g

Variations and Tips

For diabetics: Use a sugar-free pesto or make homemade pesto without added sugars to control carbohydrate content.
For allergies: Use a dairy-free pesto alternative, replacing cheese with nutritional yeast, and check for nut allergies if pesto contains nuts.
Flavor tip: Add a sprinkle of red pepper flakes for a spicy kick.

Zesty Kale & Tomato Scramble

Prep: 5 minutes   Cook: 10 minutes   Serves: 2

Ingredients:

- 4 large eggs
- 1 cup (70g) kale, chopped
- 1/2 cup (80g) cherry tomatoes, halved
- 1 tbsp (15 ml) olive oil
- 1/2 tsp (2g) ground turmeric (anti-inflammatory boost)
- 1/4 tsp (1g) ground black pepper
- Salt to taste
- Fresh parsley for garnish (optional)

Instructions:

1. **Sauté kale and tomatoes**: Heat olive oil in a pan over medium heat. Add chopped kale and cherry tomatoes, sauté for 3-4 minutes until softened.
2. **Whisk eggs**: In a bowl, whisk the eggs with turmeric, black pepper, and salt.
3. **Cook eggs**: Pour the whisked eggs into the pan with the kale and tomatoes. Gently stir and cook for 3-4 minutes until the eggs are scrambled and cooked through.
4. **Serve**: Garnish with fresh parsley if desired and serve immediately.

Nutritional Facts (Per Serving):
Calories: 200 | Carbs: 5g | Protein: 14g | Fat: 14g |Sugar: 3g

Variations and Tips

For diabetics: Reduce or omit the tomatoes if necessary to control sugar intake, or use green leafy vegetables like spinach instead.
For allergies: No changes needed, as this recipe is already dairy-free and gluten-free.
Flavor tip: Add a squeeze of fresh lemon juice at the end to enhance the flavors

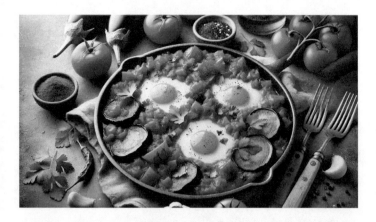

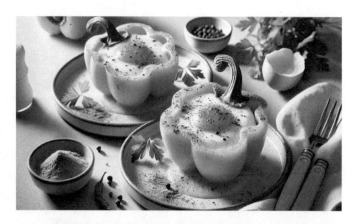

Eggplant Tomato Shakshuka Delight

Prep: 10 minutes   Cook: 20 minutes   Serves: 2

Ingredients:

- 1 small eggplant (200g), diced
- 1 cup (240g) crushed tomatoes
- 1/2 onion (60g), finely chopped
- 1 clove garlic, minced
- 2 tbsp (30 ml) olive oil
- 1/2 tsp (2g) ground cumin
- 1/2 tsp (2g) ground turmeric (anti-inflammatory boost)
- 1/4 tsp (1g) smoked paprika
- 4 large eggs
- Salt and pepper to taste
- Fresh cilantro or parsley for garnish

Instructions:

1. **Sauté vegetables**: Heat 1 tbsp of olive oil in a large skillet over medium heat. Add diced eggplant and cook for 5-7 minutes until softened. Set aside.
2. **Prepare sauce**: In the same skillet, add another 1 tbsp of olive oil and sauté onions and garlic until fragrant, about 3 minutes. Add crushed tomatoes, cumin, turmeric, paprika, salt, and pepper. Simmer for 5 minutes.
3. **Combine and cook eggs**: Return the eggplant to the skillet with the tomato sauce. Make four wells in the sauce and crack the eggs into each well. Cover and cook for 5-7 minutes, or until eggs reach your preferred doneness.
4. **Serve**: Garnish with fresh cilantro or parsley and serve immediately.

Nutritional Facts (Per Serving):
Calories: 250 | Carbs: 12g | Protein: 12g | Fat: 18g | Sugar: 6g

Variations and Tips

For diabetics: Reduce or omit the tomatoes and replace with diced bell peppers to lower the sugar content.
For allergies: Ensure the dish is dairy-free or replace olive oil with another suitable cooking oil for nut allergies.
Flavor tip: Add a pinch of red pepper flakes or fresh chili for extra heat.

Egg-Stuffed Bell Pepper Rings

Prep: 5 minutes   Cook: 10 minutes   Serves: 2

Ingredients:

- 2 large bell peppers, cut into 4 thick rings (about 1.5 cm each)
- 4 large eggs
- 1 tbsp (15 ml) olive oil
- 1/4 tsp (1g) ground turmeric (anti-inflammatory boost)
- 1/4 tsp (1g) ground black pepper
- Salt to taste
- Fresh parsley or chives for garnish (optional)

Instructions:

1. **Prepare the bell pepper rings**: Heat olive oil in a non-stick skillet over medium heat. Place the bell pepper rings in the skillet.
2. **Cook the eggs**: Crack one egg into each bell pepper ring. Sprinkle with turmeric, black pepper, and salt. Cook for about 3-4 minutes or until the egg whites are set, then cover the skillet and cook for another 2 minutes until the yolks reach your desired doneness.
3. **Serve**: Carefully transfer the stuffed bell pepper rings to plates and garnish with fresh parsley or chives if desired.

Nutritional Facts (Per Serving):
Calories: 180 | Carbs: 4g | Protein: 12g | Fat: 14g | Sugar: 3g

Variations and Tips

For diabetics: Bell peppers are already low in carbs, making this dish naturally suitable.
For allergies: Use avocado oil if you're allergic to olive oil, or ghee if you prefer a richer flavor.
Flavor tip: Add a pinch of smoked paprika or red pepper flakes for an extra kick of flavor

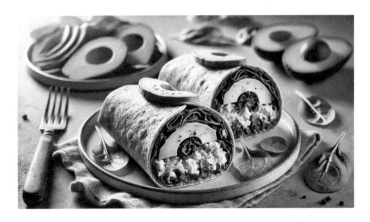

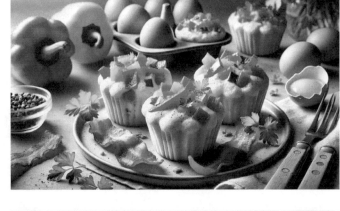

Spinach Avocado Egg Wrap

Prep: 10 minutes   Cook: 5 minutes   Serves: 2

Ingredients:

- 4 large eggs
- 1 tbsp (15 ml) olive oil
- 1 cup (30g) fresh spinach
- 1 small avocado (100g), sliced
- 1/4 tsp (1g) ground turmeric (anti-inflammatory boost)
- Salt and pepper to taste
- 2 whole grain or low-carb tortillas

Instructions:

1. **Cook spinach and eggs**: Heat olive oil in a non-stick pan over medium heat. Add spinach and cook for 1-2 minutes until wilted. In a bowl, whisk the eggs with turmeric, salt, and pepper. Pour the eggs into the pan and scramble for 3-4 minutes until fully cooked.
2. **Assemble the wraps**: Lay the tortillas flat. Divide the scrambled eggs and spinach between the two tortillas. Top with sliced avocado.
3. **Serve**: Roll the tortillas into wraps, cut in half, and serve immediately.

Nutritional Facts (Per Serving):
Calories: 320 | Carbs: 15g | Protein: 12g | Fat: 22g | Sugar: 2g

Variations and Tips

For diabetics: Use low-carb or grain-free tortillas to reduce carb content.
For allergies: Replace olive oil with avocado oil, and use gluten-free tortillas if necessary.
Flavor tip: Add a squeeze of fresh lemon juice or a sprinkle of chili flakes for extra flavor

Bell Pepper & Turkey Bacon Egg Muffins

Prep: 10 minutes   Cook: 20 minutes   Serves: 2

Ingredients:

- 4 large eggs
- 1/2 cup (60g) diced bell peppers
- 2 slices turkey bacon, chopped
- 1 tbsp (15 ml) olive oil
- 1/4 tsp (1g) ground black pepper
- 1/4 tsp (1g) ground turmeric (for anti-inflammatory benefits)
- Salt to taste
- Fresh parsley for garnish (optional)

Instructions:

1. **Preheat oven**: Preheat oven to 350°F (175°C). Lightly grease a muffin tin with olive oil.
2. **Prepare the filling**: In a pan, cook the chopped turkey bacon for 3-4 minutes until crispy. Remove from heat and set aside. Sauté diced bell peppers in the same pan for 2-3 minutes until softened.
3. **Mix the eggs**: In a bowl, whisk together the eggs, black pepper, turmeric, and salt. Stir in the cooked turkey bacon and bell peppers.
4. **Bake**: Divide the mixture evenly into 4 muffin tin cups and bake for 15-18 minutes, or until the eggs are set.
5. **Serve**: Garnish with fresh parsley and serve warm.

Nutritional Facts (Per Serving):
Calories: 200 | Carbs: 3g | Protein: 14g | Fat: 14g |Sugar: 2g

Variations and Tips

For diabetics: This recipe is already low in carbs, making it suitable.
For allergies: Ensure the turkey bacon is free of preservatives or opt for a plant-based alternative.
Flavor tip: Add a sprinkle of nutritional yeast for a cheesy flavor without dairy

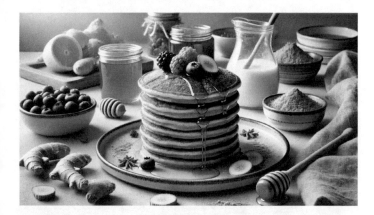

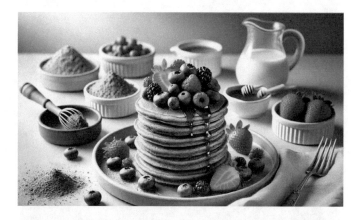

Ginger Turmeric Pancakes

Prep: 10 minutes   Cook: 10 minutes   Serves: 2

Ingredients:

- 1 cup (120g) whole wheat flour or almond flour
- 1 tsp (5g) ground turmeric (anti-inflammatory boost)
- 1/2 tsp (2g) ground ginger
- 1/2 tsp (2g) ground cinnamon
- 1 tsp (5g) baking powder

- 1 large egg
- 1/2 cup (120 ml) almond milk (or any non-dairy milk)
- 1 tbsp (15 ml) honey or maple syrup (optional)
- 1/2 tsp (2g) vanilla extract
- 1 tbsp (15 ml) olive oil or coconut oil for cooking

Instructions:

1. **Prepare the batter**: In a bowl, combine the flour, turmeric, ginger, cinnamon, and baking powder. In a separate bowl, whisk together the egg, almond milk, honey, and vanilla extract. Gradually mix the wet ingredients into the dry ingredients until a smooth batter forms.
2. **Cook the pancakes**: Heat a non-stick skillet over medium heat and add olive oil or coconut oil. Pour 1/4 cup of batter into the pan and cook for 2-3 minutes on each side until golden brown.
3. **Serve**: Stack the pancakes and serve with a drizzle of honey or maple syrup (optional) and garnish with fresh fruit if desired

Nutritional Facts (Per Serving):
Calories: 220 | Carbs: 30g | Protein: 6g | Fat: 8g | Sugar: 5g

Variations and Tips

For diabetics: Omit the honey and maple syrup, or use a sugar-free alternative.
For allergies: Replace almond milk with oat milk if needed.
Flavor tip: Add a pinch of black pepper to enhance the absorption of turmeric's anti-inflammatory benefits.

Matcha Green Tea Pancakes with Berries

Prep: 10 minutes   Cook: 10 minutes   Serves: 2

Ingredients:

- 1 cup (120g) whole wheat flour or almond flour
- 1 tsp (5g) matcha green tea powder 1 tsp (5g) baking powder
- 1 large egg
- 1/2 cup (120 ml) almond milk

- 1 tbsp (15 ml) honey or maple syrup (optional)
- 1/2 tsp (2g) vanilla extract
- 1/2 cup (75g) fresh mixed berries
- 1 tbsp (15 ml) olive oil or coconut oil for cooking

Instructions:

1. **Prepare the batter**: In a bowl, combine the flour, matcha powder, and baking powder. In a separate bowl, whisk together the egg, almond milk, honey, and vanilla extract. Gradually mix the wet ingredients into the dry ingredients until a smooth batter forms.
2. **Cook the pancakes**: Heat a non-stick skillet over medium heat and add olive oil or coconut oil. Pour 1/4 cup of batter into the pan and cook for 2-3 minutes on each side until golden brown.
3. **Serve**: Stack the pancakes and top with fresh berries. Drizzle with honey or maple syrup if desired.

Nutritional Facts (Per Serving):
Calories: 240 | Carbs: 40g | Protein: 7g | Fat: 8g | Sugar: 10g
Variations and Tips

For diabetics: Use unsweetened berries and omit maple syrup.
For allergies: Replace oat milk with almond or coconut milk.
Flavor tip: Add a few crushed walnuts or almonds for a crunchy texture.

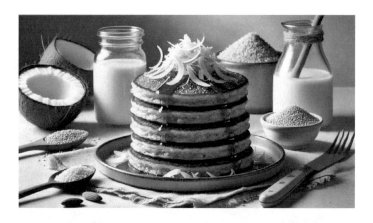

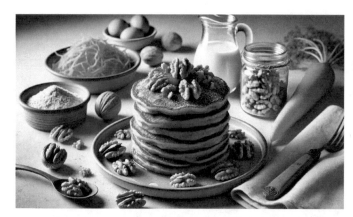

Coconut Quinoa Protein Pancakes

Prep: 10 minutes   Cook: 10 minutes   Serves: 2

Ingredients:

- 1/2 cup (60g) cooked quinoa
- 1/4 cup (30g) coconut flour
- 2 large eggs
- 1/2 cup (120 ml) almond milk (or any non-dairy milk)
- 1 tbsp (15 ml) coconut oil
- 1/2 tsp (2g) baking powder
- 1 tbsp (15 ml) maple syrup (optional)
- 1/2 tsp (2g) vanilla extract
- 1 tbsp (15g) shredded coconut (for topping, optional)

Instructions:

1. **Prepare the batter**: In a bowl, combine the cooked quinoa, coconut flour, baking powder, eggs, almond milk, maple syrup, and vanilla extract. Mix until smooth.
2. **Cook the pancakes**: Heat a non-stick skillet over medium heat and add coconut oil. Pour 1/4 cup of batter onto the skillet and cook for 2-3 minutes on each side until golden brown.
3. **Serve**: Stack the pancakes and top with shredded coconut or additional maple syrup if desired

Nutritional Facts (Per Serving):
Calories: 240 | Carbs: 25g | Protein: 8g | Fat: 12g | Sugar: 6g

Variations and Tips

For diabetics: Omit the maple syrup or use a sugar-free alternative.
For allergies: Replace almond milk with oat or coconut milk if necessary.
Flavor tip: Add a sprinkle of cinnamon or nutmeg to the batter for extra warmth and flavor

Carrot Cake Pancakes with Walnuts

Prep: 10 minutes   Cook: 10 minutes   Serves: 2

Ingredients:

- 1/2 cup (60g) grated carrots
- 1/2 cup (60g) whole wheat or almond flour
- 1/4 cup (30g) chopped walnuts
- 2 large eggs
- 1/2 cup (120 ml) almond milk (or any non-dairy milk)
- 1 tbsp (15 ml) olive oil or coconut oil
- 1 tsp (5g) ground cinnamon
- 1/2 tsp (2g) ground ginger
- 1 tsp (5g) baking powder
- 1 tbsp (15 ml) maple syrup (optional)
- 1/2 tsp (2g) vanilla extract

Instructions:

1. **Prepare the batter**: In a bowl, mix the grated carrots, flour, cinnamon, ginger, baking powder, eggs, almond milk, and vanilla extract. Stir in the chopped walnuts.
2. **Cook the pancakes**: Heat olive oil or coconut oil in a non-stick skillet over medium heat. Pour 1/4 cup of batter into the skillet and cook for 2-3 minutes on each side until golden brown.
3. **Serve**: Stack the pancakes and drizzle with maple syrup if desired

Nutritional Facts (Per Serving):
Calories: 270 | Carbs: 30g | Protein: 8g | Fat: 14g | Sugar: 7g

Variations and Tips

For diabetics: Omit the maple syrup or use a sugar-free sweetener.
For allergies: Replace almond milk with coconut or oat milk.
Flavor tip: Add a pinch of nutmeg or cardamom for a richer spice profile

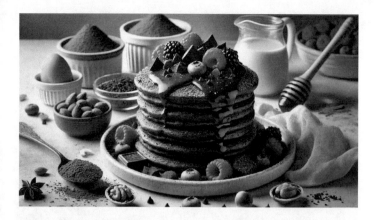

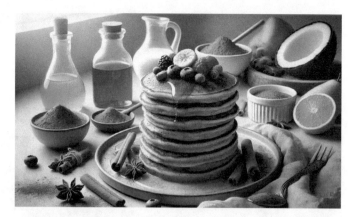

Chocolate Hazelnut Superfood Pancakes

Prep: 10 minutes   Cook: 10 minutes   Serves: 2

Ingredients:

- 1/2 cup (60g) almond flour
- 2 tbsp (15g) cocoa powder (unsweetened)
- 1/4 cup (30g) ground hazelnuts
- 1 large egg
- 1/2 cup (120ml) almond milk (or any non-dairy milk)
- 1 tbsp (15ml) maple syrup (optional)
- 1/2 tsp (2g) baking powder
- 1 tsp (5g) vanilla extract
- 1 tbsp (15ml) olive oil or coconut oil for cooking
- 1 tbsp (15g) dark chocolate chips (optional)
- Fresh berries for serving (optional)

Instructions:

1. **Prepare the batter**: In a bowl, whisk together almond flour, cocoa powder, ground hazelnuts, and baking powder. In a separate bowl, whisk together the egg, almond milk, maple syrup, and vanilla extract. Slowly add the wet ingredients to the dry and stir until combined.
2. **Cook the pancakes**: Heat a non-stick skillet over medium heat and add olive oil or coconut oil. Pour 1/4 cup of batter into the pan and cook for 2-3 minutes on each side until golden brown.
3. **Serve**: Stack the pancakes and top with dark chocolate chips and fresh berries, if desired.

Nutritional Facts (Per Serving):
Calories: 280 | Carbs: 22g | Protein: 10g | Fat: 18g | Sugar: 8g

Variations and Tips

For diabetics: Omit the maple syrup and use a sugar-free chocolate alternative.
For allergies: Replace almond milk with coconut or oat milk, and ensure chocolate is dairy-free.
Flavor tip: Add a sprinkle of cinnamon or nutmeg to enhance the flavor

Golden Cinnamon Spice Pancakes

Prep: 10 minutes   Cook: 10 minutes   Serves: 2

Ingredients:

- 1/2 cup (60g) whole wheat flour or almond flour
- 1 tsp (5g) ground cinnamon
- 1/2 tsp (2g) ground turmeric (anti-inflammatory)
- 1/2 tsp (2g) ground ginger
- 1 tsp (5g) baking powder
- 1 large egg
- 1/2 cup (120ml) coconut milk (or any non-dairy milk)
- 1 tbsp (15ml) olive oil or coconut oil for cooking
- 1 tbsp (15ml) maple syrup (optional)
- 1/2 tsp (2g) vanilla extract

Instructions:

1. **Prepare the batter**: In a bowl, whisk together the flour, cinnamon, turmeric, ginger, and baking powder. In a separate bowl, whisk together the egg, coconut milk, maple syrup, and vanilla extract. Combine wet and dry ingredients until smooth.
2. **Cook the pancakes**: Heat a non-stick skillet over medium heat and add olive oil or coconut oil. Pour 1/4 cup of batter into the pan and cook for 2-3 minutes on each side until golden brown.
3. **Serve**: Stack the pancakes and serve with fresh fruit or a drizzle of honey, if desired

Nutritional Facts (Per Serving):
Calories: 240 | Carbs: 26g | Protein: 8g | Fat: 12g | Sugar: 6g

Variations and Tips

For diabetics: Omit the maple syrup or use a sugar-free sweetener.
For allergies: Replace coconut milk with almond or oat milk if needed.
Flavor tip: Add a pinch of black pepper to enhance the absorption of turmeric's anti-inflammatory benefits

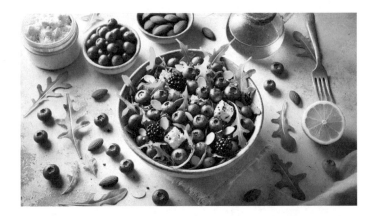

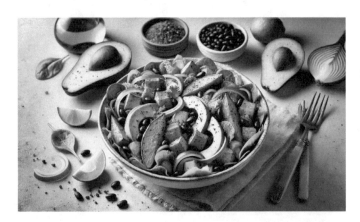

Blueberry Almond Arugula Salad with Goat Cheese

Prep: 10 minutes	Cook: N/A	Serves: 2

Ingredients:

- 2 cups (60g) arugula
- 1/2 cup (75g) fresh blueberries
- 1/4 cup (30g) sliced almonds, toasted
- 1/4 cup (30g) crumbled goat cheese
- 1 tbsp (15ml) olive oil
- 1 tbsp (15ml) lemon juice
- 1 tsp (5ml) honey (optional)
- Salt and pepper to taste

Instructions:

1. **Prepare the salad**: In a large bowl, combine arugula, blueberries, toasted almonds, and crumbled goat cheese.
2. **Make the dressing**: In a small bowl, whisk together olive oil, lemon juice, honey (if using), salt, and pepper.
3. **Assemble the salad**: Drizzle the dressing over the salad and toss gently to combine

Nutritional Facts (Per Serving):
Calories: 220 | Carbs: 14g | Protein: 7g | Fat: 17g | Sugar: 8g

Variations and Tips

For diabetics: Omit the honey or use a sugar-free alternative.
For allergies: Replace almonds with sunflower seeds for a nut-free option.
Flavor tip: Add a handful of fresh mint leaves for a refreshing twist

Roasted Sweet Potato & Black Bean Power Salad

Prep: 10 minutes	Cook: 20 minutes	Serves: 2

Ingredients:

- 1 medium sweet potato (200g), diced
- 1/2 cup (120g) black beans, cooked or canned (rinsed and drained)
- 2 cups (60g) mixed greens
- 1/2 avocado (75g), diced
- 1/4 cup (30g) red onion, thinly sliced
- 1 tbsp (15ml) olive oil
- 1/2 tsp (2g) ground cumin
- 1 tbsp (15ml) lime juice
- 1 tbsp (15ml) olive oil (for dressing)
- Salt and pepper to taste

Instructions:

1. **Roast the sweet potato**: Preheat oven to 400°F (200°C). Toss the diced sweet potato with olive oil, cumin, salt, and pepper. Roast for 20 minutes, or until tender and slightly crispy.
2. **Prepare the salad**: In a large bowl, combine mixed greens, black beans, avocado, and red onion.
3. **Make the dressing**: In a small bowl, whisk together lime juice, olive oil, salt, and pepper.
4. **Assemble the salad**: Add the roasted sweet potatoes to the salad, drizzle with the dressing, and toss to combine

Nutritional Facts (Per Serving):
Calories: 320 | Carbs: 38g | Protein: 7g | Fat: 18g | Sugar: 6g

Variations and Tips

For diabetics: Reduce the portion of sweet potatoes or replace with roasted cauliflower for a lower-carb option.
For allergies: Ensure all ingredients are nut-free, or substitute avocado with olives if allergic to avocados.
Flavor tip: Add a sprinkle of chili flakes for a spicy kick

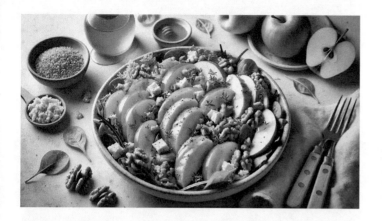

Honey Dijon Chicken & Apple Salad

Prep: 10 minutes   Cook: 15 minutes   Serves: 2

Ingredients:

- 2 chicken breasts (about 300g)
- 1 tbsp (15 ml) olive oil
- 1/4 tsp (1g) ground black pepper
- Salt to taste
- 1 medium apple (100g), sliced
- 2 cups (60g) mixed greens
- 1/4 cup (30g) walnuts, chopped
- 1/4 cup (30g) crumbled feta cheese (optional)

Dressing:

- 1 tbsp (15 ml) Dijon mustard
- 1 tbsp (15 ml) honey
- 2 tbsp (30 ml) olive oil
- 1 tbsp (15 ml) apple cider vinegar
- 1/4 tsp (1g) ground turmeric
- Salt and pepper to taste

Instructions:

1. **Cook the chicken**: Heat 1 tbsp of olive oil in a skillet over medium heat. Season chicken breasts with salt and black pepper, and cook for 6-7 minutes per side or until fully cooked. Let rest for 5 minutes, then slice.
2. **Prepare the salad**: In a large bowl, combine mixed greens, apple slices, walnuts, and feta cheese (if using).
3. **Make the dressing**: In a small bowl, whisk together Dijon mustard, honey, olive oil, apple cider vinegar, turmeric, salt, and pepper.
4. **Assemble the salad**: Add sliced chicken to the salad, drizzle with dressing, and toss to combine

Nutritional Facts (Per Serving):
Calories: 420 | Carbs: 18g | Protein: 28g | Fat: 25g | Sugar: 10g

Variations and Tips

For diabetics: Reduce or omit the honey in the dressing, or use a sugar-free alternative.
For allergies: Replace walnuts with pumpkin seeds for a nut-free option.
Flavor tip: Add a sprinkle of cinnamon to the apple slices for a sweet and spicy flavor boost

Grilled Chicken & Avocado Romaine Crunch Salad

Prep: 10 minutes   Cook: 15 minutes   Serves: 2

Ingredients:

- 2 chicken breasts (about 300g)
- 1 tbsp (15 ml) olive oil
- 1 avocado (100g), diced
- 3 cups (90g) romaine lettuce, chopped
- 1/2 cup (75g) cherry tomatoes, halved
- 1/4 cup (30g) red onion, thinly sliced
- 1 tbsp (15 ml) lemon juice
- 1 tbsp (15 ml) olive oil for dressing
- 1/4 tsp (1g) ground black pepper
- Salt to taste

Instructions:

1. **Grill the chicken**: Heat a grill pan or outdoor grill to medium-high heat. Brush chicken breasts with olive oil, season with salt and pepper, and grill for 6-7 minutes on each side until fully cooked. Let rest for 5 minutes, then slice.
2. **Prepare the salad**: In a large bowl, toss romaine lettuce, avocado, cherry tomatoes, and red onion.
3. **Make the dressing**: In a small bowl, whisk together lemon juice, olive oil, black pepper, and salt.
4. **Assemble the salad**: Add the grilled chicken slices to the salad, drizzle with dressing, and toss to combine

Nutritional Facts (Per Serving):
Calories: 380 | Carbs:12g | Protein:30g | Fat: 23g | Sugar: 3g

Variations and Tips

For diabetics: This recipe is already low in carbs, making it suitable.
For allergies: Ensure the chicken is free from preservatives or additives, or replace it with a plant-based protein like grilled tofu.
Flavor tip: Add a few fresh basil leaves for an aromatic touch

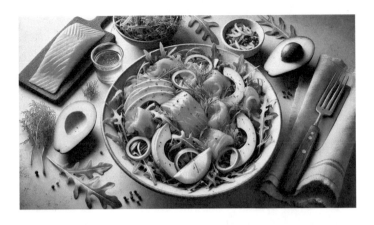

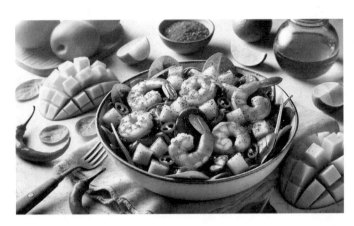

Smoked Salmon & Avocado Arugula Salad

Prep: 10 minutes   **Cook: N/A**   **Serves: 2**

Ingredients:

- 2 cups (60g) arugula
- 100g smoked salmon, sliced
- 1 avocado (100g), sliced
- 1/4 cup (30g) red onion, thinly sliced
- 1 tbsp (15ml) olive oil
- 1 tbsp (15ml) lemon juice
- 1 tsp (5g) Dijon mustard
- Salt and pepper to taste
- Fresh dill for garnish (optional)

Instructions:

1. **Prepare the salad**: In a large bowl, combine arugula, smoked salmon, avocado, and red onion.
2. **Make the dressing**: In a small bowl, whisk together olive oil, lemon juice, Dijon mustard, salt, and pepper.
3. **Assemble the salad**: Drizzle the dressing over the salad and toss gently to combine. Garnish with fresh dill if desired.

Nutritional Facts (Per Serving):
Calories: 310 | Carbs: 9g | Protein: 15g | Fat: 25g | Sugar: 2g

Variations and Tips

For diabetics: This recipe is naturally low in carbs and suitable as-is.
For allergies: Ensure the smoked salmon is free of added preservatives, or replace with grilled tofu for a plant-based option.
Flavor tip: Add a sprinkle of capers for an extra burst of flavor

Spicy Shrimp & Mango Spinach Salad

Prep: 10 minutes   **Cook: 5 minutes**   **Serves: 2**

Ingredients:

- 200g shrimp, peeled and deveined
- 1 tbsp (15ml) olive oil
- 1/2 tsp (2g) chili powder
- 1/2 tsp (2g) paprika
- 1/2 mango (100g), diced
- 2 cups (60g) fresh spinach
- 1/4 cup (30g) red bell pepper, thinly sliced
- 1 tbsp (15ml) lime juice
- 1 tbsp (15ml) olive oil (for dressing)
- Salt and pepper to taste

Instructions:

1. **Cook the shrimp**: Heat 1 tbsp of olive oil in a skillet over medium heat. Season shrimp with chili powder, paprika, salt, and pepper. Cook for 2-3 minutes on each side until shrimp are opaque and cooked through.
2. **Prepare the salad**: In a large bowl, combine spinach, mango, and red bell pepper.
3. **Make the dressing**: In a small bowl, whisk together lime juice, olive oil, salt, and pepper.
4. **Assemble the salad**: Add the cooked shrimp to the salad, drizzle with the dressing, and toss to combine

Nutritional Facts (Per Serving):
Calories: 290 | Carbs:14g | Protein:20g | Fat: 18g | Sugar: 8g

Variations and Tips

For diabetics: Use less mango or replace with strawberries to reduce sugar content.
For allergies: Replace shrimp with grilled chicken or tempeh for a seafood-free option.
Flavor tip: Add a sprinkle of crushed red pepper flakes for extra heat

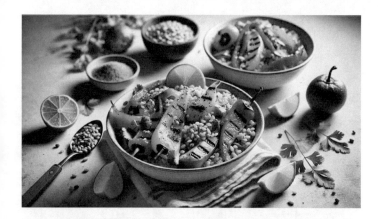

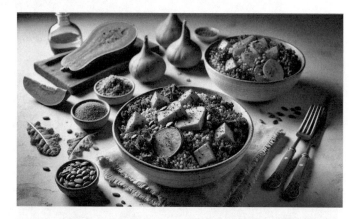

Zesty Lime Barley Bowl with Grilled Peppers

Prep: 10 minutes   Cook: 25 minutes   Serves: 2

Ingredients:

- 1/2 cup (100g) barley
- 1 cup (240ml) water or vegetable broth
- 1 red bell pepper (120g), sliced
- 1 yellow bell pepper (120g), sliced
- 1 tbsp (15ml) olive oil
- 1 tbsp (15ml) lime juice
- 1/2 tsp (2g) ground cumin
- 1/2 tsp (2g) ground coriander
- 1/4 cup (30g) chopped fresh cilantro
- Salt and pepper to taste
- Lime wedges for serving

Instructions:

1. **Cook the barley**: In a medium saucepan, combine barley and water or vegetable broth. Bring to a boil, reduce heat, and simmer for 20-25 minutes, or until the barley is tender. Drain any excess liquid.
2. **Grill the peppers**: While the barley is cooking, heat 1 tbsp of olive oil in a grill pan over medium heat. Add sliced red and yellow bell peppers, season with cumin, coriander, salt, and pepper, and grill for 4-5 minutes, turning occasionally until tender and slightly charred.
3. **Assemble the bowl**: In a large bowl, combine the cooked barley, grilled peppers, lime juice, and chopped cilantro. Toss gently to combine.
4. **Serve**: Divide into two bowls and serve with lime wedges for an extra zesty kick

Nutritional Facts (Per Serving):
Calories: 250 | Carbs: 38g | Protein: 5g | Fat: 9g | Sugar: 4g

Variations and Tips

For diabetics: Replace barley with quinoa for a lower glycemic index.
For allergies: Ensure the barley is gluten-free certified or substitute with brown rice.
Flavor tip: Add a sprinkle of chili flakes for a spicy touch

Sweet Potato & Kale Freekeh Bowl

Prep: 10 minutes   Cook: 30 minutes   Serves: 2

Ingredients:

- 1/2 cup (100g) freekeh
- 1 cup (240ml) water or vegetable broth
- 1 medium sweet potato (200g), diced
- 2 cups (60g) kale, chopped
- 1 tbsp (15ml) olive oil
- 1/2 tsp (2g) ground cumin
- 1/4 tsp (1g) ground cinnamon
- 1 tbsp (15ml) lemon juice
- 1 tbsp (15g) pumpkin seeds
- Salt and pepper to taste

Instructions:

1. **Cook the freekeh**: Boil freekeh in water or broth for 20-25 minutes until tender. Drain and set aside.
2. **Roast the sweet potato**: Toss diced sweet potato with olive oil, cumin, cinnamon, salt, and pepper. Roast at 400°F (200°C) for 20-25 minutes.
3. **Sauté the kale**: Heat olive oil in a skillet and sauté kale with salt for 3-5 minutes until wilted.
4. **Assemble the bowl**: Combine freekeh, sweet potato, and kale in a bowl. Drizzle with lemon juice and top with pumpkin seeds. Serve warm.

Nutritional Facts (Per Serving):
Calories: 340 | Carbs: 50g | Protein: 9g | Fat: 12g | Sugar: 8g

Variations and Tips

For diabetics: Replace freekeh with quinoa or a lower glycemic grain like buckwheat.
For allergies: Substitute pumpkin seeds with sunflower seeds for a nut-free option.
Flavor tip: Add a pinch of chili flakes for extra heat, or top with a dollop of tahini for a creamy texture

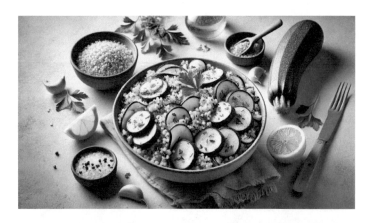

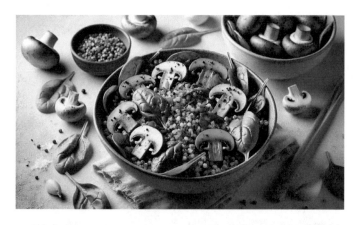

Lemon Garlic Bulgur Bowl with Zucchini

Prep: 10 minutes   Cook: 20 minutes   Serves: 2

Ingredients:

- 1/2 cup (100g) bulgur
- 1 cup (240ml) water or vegetable broth
- 1 medium zucchini (150g), sliced
- 1 tbsp (15ml) olive oil
- 1 garlic clove, minced
- 1 tbsp (15ml) lemon juice
- 1/4 tsp (1g) ground black pepper
- Salt to taste
- 1 tbsp (15g) chopped fresh parsley for garnish

Instructions:

1. **Cook the bulgur**: In a saucepan, bring water or broth to a boil. Add bulgur, reduce heat, cover, and simmer for 12-15 minutes until the bulgur is tender and the liquid is absorbed. Fluff with a fork.
2. **Sauté the zucchini**: In a skillet, heat olive oil over medium heat. Add sliced zucchini and cook for 4-5 minutes until slightly browned. Add minced garlic and sauté for 1 more minute.
3. **Assemble the bowl**: Combine the cooked bulgur and sautéed zucchini in a large bowl. Drizzle with lemon juice, season with salt and pepper, and toss to combine. Garnish with fresh parsley.
4. **Serve**: Divide between two bowls and serve warm

Nutritional Facts (Per Serving):
Calories: 220 | Carbs: 35g | Protein: 5g | Fat: 8g | Sugar: 3g

Variations and Tips

For diabetics: Replace bulgur with quinoa for a lower glycemic index.
For allergies: Substitute bulgur with buckwheat for a gluten-free option.
Flavor tip: Add a pinch of chili flakes for extra heat

Toasted Buckwheat Bowl with Mushrooms & Spinach

Prep: 10 minutes   Cook: 20 minutes   Serves: 2

Ingredients:

- 1/2 cup (100g) buckwheat
- 1 cup (240ml) vegetable broth
- 1 tbsp (15ml) olive oil
- 100g mushrooms, sliced
- 2 cups (60g) fresh spinach
- 1 garlic clove, minced
- 1 tbsp (15ml) soy sauce or tamari (for gluten-free)
- 1/4 tsp (1g) ground black pepper
- Salt to taste

Instructions:

1. **Toast buckwheat**: Toast buckwheat in a dry skillet for 3-4 minutes.
2. **Cook buckwheat**: Simmer buckwheat in broth for 12-15 minutes until tender.
3. **Sauté mushrooms and spinach**: Sauté mushrooms for 5-6 minutes, add garlic and spinach, and cook until wilted.
4. **Assemble the bowl**: Combine buckwheat, mushrooms, and spinach. Add soy sauce, salt, and pepper.
5. **Serve**: Divide between two bowls and serve warm

Nutritional Facts (Per Serving):
Calories: 250 | Carbs: 35g | Protein: 8g | Fat: 9g | Sugar: 2g

Variations and Tips

For diabetics: This recipe is already low glycemic and suitable as is.
For allergies: Ensure the soy sauce is gluten-free or replace with coconut aminos.
Flavor tip: Add a sprinkle of sesame seeds for a nutty flavor and extra crunch

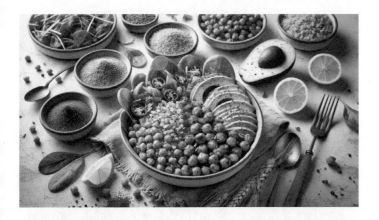

Crispy Chickpea & Barley Buddha Bowl

Prep: 10 minutes   Cook: 30 minutes   Serves: 2

Ingredients:

- 1/2 cup (100g) barley
- 1 cup (240ml) vegetable broth or water
- 1 can (400g) chickpeas, drained and rinsed
- 1 tbsp (15ml) olive oil
- 1 tsp (5g) smoked paprika
- 1/2 tsp (2g) cumin
- 1/4 tsp (1g) garlic powder
- 2 cups (60g) mixed greens
- 1/2 avocado (75g), sliced
- 1 tbsp (15ml) lemon juice
- Salt and pepper to taste

Instructions:

1. **Cook barley**: Boil broth or water, add barley, simmer for 25-30 minutes until tender. Fluff with a fork.
2. **Roast chickpeas**: Toss chickpeas with olive oil, paprika, cumin, garlic powder, salt, and pepper. Roast at 400°F (200°C) for 20-25 minutes until crispy.
3. **Assemble**: Divide barley and greens into bowls. Top with chickpeas, avocado, and drizzle with lemon juice.
4. **Serve**: Season to taste and enjoy

Nutritional Facts (Per Serving):
Calories: 380 | Carbs: 50g | Protein: 12g | Fat: 15g | Sugar: 3g

Variations and Tips

For diabetics: Replace barley with quinoa or buckwheat for a lower glycemic option.
For allergies: Replace chickpeas with roasted tofu or tempeh for a legume-free option.
Flavor tip: Add a sprinkle of chili flakes or fresh herbs for extra flavor.

Avocado & Sriracha Millet Bowl

Prep: 10 minutes   Cook: 20 minutes   Serves: 2

Ingredients:

- 1/2 cup (100g) millet
- 1 cup (240ml) vegetable broth or water
- 1 avocado (100g), sliced
- 1 tbsp (15ml) sriracha
- 1 tbsp (15ml) olive oil
- 1 tbsp (15ml) lime juice
- 1/4 cup (30g) red cabbage, shredded
- 1/4 cup (30g) carrots, julienned
- 1 tbsp (15g) sesame seeds
- Salt and pepper to taste

Instructions:

1. **Cook millet**: Boil broth or water, add millet, simmer for 15-20 minutes until tender. Fluff with a fork.
2. **Prepare veggies**: Divide millet into bowls, top with avocado, cabbage, and carrots.
3. **Assemble**: Drizzle with sriracha, olive oil, and lime juice. Sprinkle with sesame seeds.
4. **Serve**: Mix and enjoy

Nutritional Facts (Per Serving):
Calories: 350 | Carbs: 45g | Protein: 8g | Fat: 15g | Sugar: 4g

Variations and Tips

For diabetics: Reduce the portion of millet or replace with cauliflower rice for a low-carb option.
For allergies: Replace sesame seeds with sunflower seeds for a nut-free version.
Flavor tip: Add a pinch of smoked paprika or fresh cilantro for extra flavor

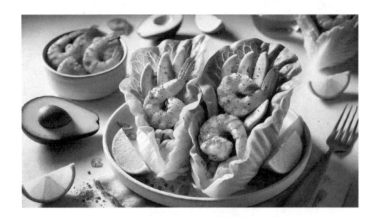

Chili-Lime Shrimp & Avocado Lettuce Wrap

Prep: 10 minutes   **Cook: 5 minutes**   **Serves: 2**

Ingredients:

- 200g shrimp, peeled and deveined
- 1 tbsp (15ml) olive oil
- 1 tsp chili powder
- 1 tbsp (15ml) lime juice
- 1/2 avocado (75g), sliced
- 4 large lettuce leaves (for wrapping)
- Salt and pepper to taste

Instructions:

1. **Cook the shrimp**: Heat olive oil in a skillet over medium heat. Add shrimp, chili powder, salt, and pepper. Cook for 2-3 minutes on each side until cooked through. Drizzle with lime juice.
2. **Assemble the wraps**: Place shrimp and avocado slices onto each lettuce leaf. Wrap and serve.

Nutritional Facts (Per Serving):
Calories: 220 | Carbs: 5g | Protein: 18g | Fat: 15g | Sugar: 1g

Variations and Tips

For diabetics: This recipe is already low in carbs, no changes needed.
For allergies: Replace shrimp with grilled chicken for a seafood-free option.
Flavor tip: Add fresh cilantro or a sprinkle of smoked paprika for extra flavor

Smoked Salmon & Cucumber Collard Wrap

Prep: 10 minutes   **Cook: N/A**   **Serves: 2**

Ingredients:

- 100g smoked salmon, thinly sliced
- 1/2 cucumber (75g), sliced
- 4 large collard green leaves (for wrapping)
- 1 tbsp (15ml) lemon juice
- 1 tbsp (15ml) olive oil
- 1 tbsp (15g) capers (optional)
- Salt and pepper to taste

Instructions:

1. **Assemble the wraps**: Place smoked salmon, cucumber slices, and capers (if using) onto collard green leaves. Drizzle with lemon juice and olive oil.
2. **Wrap and serve**: Roll the collard leaves tightly and serve fresh

Nutritional Facts (Per Serving):
Calories: 200 | Carbs: 4g | Protein: 14g | Fat: 13g | Sugar: 1g

Variations and Tips

For diabetics: This recipe is low in carbs, suitable as is.
For allergies: Replace smoked salmon with turkey slices for a fish-free option.
Flavor tip: Add a spread of avocado or mustard for extra creaminess.

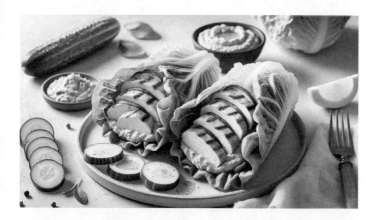

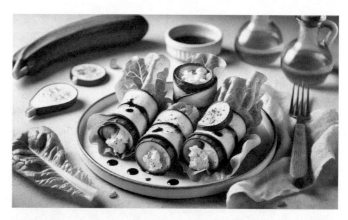

Grilled Chicken & Hummus Lettuce Wrap

Prep: 10 minutes **Cook: 10 minutes** **Serves: 2**

Ingredients:

- 200g grilled chicken breast, sliced
- 4 tbsp (60g) hummus
- 4 large lettuce leaves (for wrapping)
- 1/2 cucumber (75g), sliced
- 1 tbsp (15ml) olive oil
- 1 tbsp (15ml) lemon juice
- Salt and pepper to taste

Instructions:

1. **Grill the chicken**: Season chicken with salt, pepper, and olive oil. Grill over medium heat for 5-7 minutes per side until fully cooked. Slice into strips.
2. **Assemble the wraps**: Spread hummus on each lettuce leaf, add grilled chicken slices and cucumber. Drizzle with lemon juice.
3. **Serve**: Wrap tightly and serve fresh.

Nutritional Facts (Per Serving):
Calories: 290 | Carbs: 8g | Protein: 30g | Fat: 16g | Sugar: 1g

Variations and Tips

For diabetics: This recipe is already low in carbs, suitable as is.
For allergies: Ensure hummus is nut-free if you have a sesame allergy, or use an alternative spread like avocado
Flavor tip: Add fresh herbs like parsley or cilantro for extra freshness

Zucchini & Goat Cheese Lettuce Wrap

Prep: 10 minutes **Cook:5 minutes** **Serves: 2**

Ingredients:

- 1 medium zucchini (150g), thinly sliced
- 4 tbsp (60g) goat cheese
- 4 large lettuce leaves (for wrapping)
- 1 tbsp (15ml) olive oil
- 1 tbsp (15ml) balsamic vinegar
- Salt and pepper to taste

Instructions:

1. **Sauté zucchini**: Heat olive oil in a skillet over medium heat. Sauté zucchini slices for 2-3 minutes until tender. Season with salt and pepper.
2. **Assemble the wraps**: Spread goat cheese on each lettuce leaf, add sautéed zucchini slices. Drizzle with balsamic vinegar.
3. **Serve**: Wrap and enjoy

Nutritional Facts (Per Serving):
Calories: 220 | Carbs: 6g | Protein: 8g | Fat: 18g | Sugar: 3g

Variations and Tips

For diabetics: This recipe is naturally low in carbs, no changes needed.
For allergies: Swap out goat cheese with a dairy-free cheese alternative if lactose intolerant
Flavor tip: Add a sprinkle of pine nuts or fresh basil for more texture and flavor.

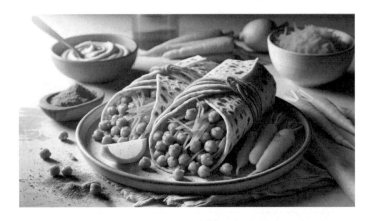

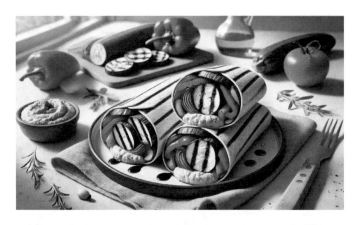

Curried Chickpea & Carrot Wrap

Prep: 10 minutes   Cook: 5 minutes   Serves: 2

Ingredients:

- 1 can (400g) chickpeas, drained and rinsed
- 1 medium carrot (100g), grated
- 2 tbsp (30ml) olive oil
- 1 tbsp (15g) curry powder
- 2 large whole wheat wraps
- 1 tbsp (15ml) lemon juice
- 1/4 cup (60g) hummus
- Salt and pepper to taste

Instructions:

1. **Cook the chickpeas**: Heat olive oil in a pan over medium heat. Add chickpeas, curry powder, salt, and pepper. Cook for 4-5 minutes, stirring occasionally. Add grated carrot and cook for 1 minute.
2. **Assemble the wraps**: Spread hummus on each wrap, top with curried chickpeas and carrot mixture. Drizzle with lemon juice.
3. **Serve**: Roll up the wraps and serve.

Nutritional Facts (Per Serving):
Calories: 350 | Carbs: 45g | Protein: 10g | Fat: 15g | Sugar: 6g

Variations and Tips

For diabetics: Use low-carb wraps or lettuce leaves instead of whole wheat wraps.
For allergies: Ensure the hummus is free from any nuts or sesame if needed, or use a different spread like avocado
Flavor tip: Add fresh cilantro or a pinch of chili flakes for extra flavor

Grilled Veggie & Hummus Wrap

Prep: 10 minutes   Cook: 10 minutes   Serves: 2

Ingredients:

- 1 zucchini (150g), sliced
- 1 red bell pepper (120g), sliced
- 1/2 red onion (50g), sliced
- 2 tbsp (30ml) olive oil
- 4 tbsp (60g) hummus
- 2 large whole wheat wraps
- 1 tbsp (15ml) balsamic vinegar
- Salt and pepper to taste

Instructions:

1. **Grill the veggies**: Heat a grill or grill pan over medium heat. Toss the zucchini, bell pepper, and onion with olive oil, salt, and pepper. Grill for 8-10 minutes until tender.
2. **Assemble the wraps**: Spread hummus on each wrap, add the grilled veggies, and drizzle with balsamic vinegar.
3. **Serve**: Roll up the wraps and enjoy

Nutritional Facts (Per Serving):
Calories: 300 | Carbs: 40g | Protein: 8g | Fat: 14g | Sugar: 7g

Variations and Tips

For diabetics: Use low-carb wraps or lettuce leaves instead of whole wheat wraps.
For allergies: Ensure the hummus is free from sesame if there is an allergy concern
Flavor tip: Add a sprinkle of fresh basil or parsley for a fresh, herbal taste

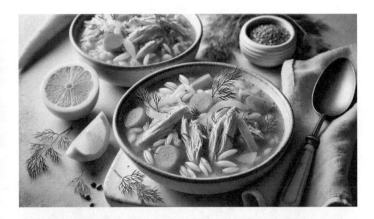

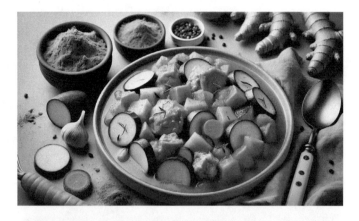

Lemon Orzo Chicken Soup with Dill

Prep: 10 minutes   Cook: 20 minutes   Serves: 2

Ingredients:

- 200g cooked chicken breast, shredded
- 1/2 cup (90g) orzo
- 1 tbsp (15ml) olive oil
- 1 garlic clove, minced
- 1/2 onion (75g), diced
- 1 carrot (80g), sliced
- 1 tbsp (15ml) lemon juice
- 4 cups (960ml) chicken broth
- 1 tbsp (10g) fresh dill, chopped
- Salt and pepper to taste

Instructions:

1. **Sauté vegetables**: Heat olive oil, add garlic, onion, and carrot. Cook 5 minutes.
2. **Cook orzo**: Add broth, bring to boil. Add orzo, cook 8-10 minutes until tender.
3. **Add chicken**: Stir in chicken, lemon juice, salt, and pepper. Cook 5 minutes.
4. **Finish**: Stir in dill, serve warm

Nutritional Facts (Per Serving):
Calories: 320 | Carbs: 35g | Protein: 25g | Fat: 9g | Sugar: 4g

Variations and Tips

For diabetics: Replace orzo with cauliflower rice or zucchini noodles for lower carbs.
For allergies: Replace orzo with gluten-free pasta for a gluten-free option.
Flavor tip: Add turmeric for extra anti-inflammatory benefits.

Turmeric Chicken & Veggie Stew

Prep: 10 minutes   Cook:30 minutes   Serves: 2

Ingredients:

- 200g chicken thighs, diced
- 1 tbsp (15ml) olive oil
- 1 garlic clove, minced
- 1 onion (100g), diced
- 1 zucchini (150g), diced
- 1 sweet potato (200g), diced
- 1 tsp (5g) turmeric
- 1/2 tsp (2g) cumin
- 4 cups (960ml) chicken broth
- 1 tbsp (15ml) lemon juice
- Salt and pepper to taste

Instructions:

1. **Brown chicken**: Heat olive oil, add chicken, cook 5-6 minutes.
2. **Add vegetables**: Add garlic, onion, zucchini, sweet potato. Cook 5 minutes.
3. **Simmer**: Add broth, turmeric, cumin. Simmer for 20 minutes until vegetables are tender.
4. **Finish**: Stir in lemon juice, serve.

Nutritional Facts (Per Serving):
Calories: 350 | Carbs:40g | Protein:28g | Fat: 10g | Sugar: 7g

Variations and Tips

For diabetics: Reduce sweet potato or replace with cauliflower for lower carbs.
For allergies: Replace chicken with tofu for a vegetarian and dairy-free option.
Flavor tip: Add fresh ginger or chili flakes for a spicier kick

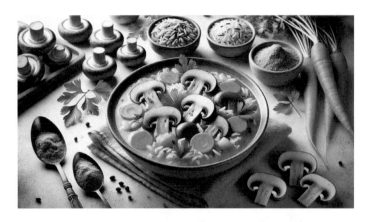

Mushroom & Wild Rice Immune Boosting Soup

Prep: 10 minutes   Cook: 35 minutes   Serves: 2

Ingredients:

- 1/2 cup (100g) wild rice
- 200g mushrooms, sliced (shiitake or cremini)
- 1 tbsp (15ml) olive oil
- 1 garlic clove, minced
- 1/2 onion (75g), diced
- 1 carrot (80g), sliced
- 4 cups (960ml) vegetable broth
- 1 tsp (5g) ground turmeric
- 1 tbsp (10g) fresh parsley, chopped
- Salt and pepper to taste

Instructions:

1. **Cook wild rice**: Boil wild rice in a pot with vegetable broth for 25-30 minutes until tender.
2. **Sauté vegetables**: In a separate pan, heat olive oil. Add garlic, onion, carrot, and mushrooms. Sauté for 5-7 minutes until softened.
3. **Combine and simmer**: Add sautéed vegetables to the pot with wild rice. Stir in turmeric, salt, and pepper. Simmer for 5 minutes.
4. **Serve**: Stir in fresh parsley and serve hot

Nutritional Facts (Per Serving):
Calories: 290 | Carbs: 45g | Protein: 8g | Fat: 9g | Sugar: 4g

Variations and Tips

For diabetics: Replace wild rice with cauliflower rice for a lower-carb option.
For allergies: Replace mushrooms with zucchini for a mushroom-free version.
Flavor tip: Add a squeeze of lemon for extra freshness.

Miso Soup with Seaweed & Tofu

Prep: 5 minutes   Cook:10 minutes   Serves: 2

Ingredients:

- 4 cups (960ml) water
- 2 tbsp (30g) miso paste
- 100g firm tofu, cubed
- 1/4 cup (10g) dried seaweed (wakame), soaked in water
- 1 tbsp (10g) green onions, chopped
- 1 tsp (5ml) soy sauce (optional)
- 1 tsp (5g) sesame seeds (optional)

Instructions:

1. **Prepare broth**: Bring water to a gentle boil, reduce heat to low. Stir in miso paste until dissolved.
2. **Add tofu and seaweed**: Add cubed tofu and soaked seaweed to the broth. Simmer for 5-7 minutes.
3. **Serve**: Garnish with green onions, soy sauce, and sesame seeds.

Nutritional Facts (Per Serving):
Calories: 130 | Carbs: 10g | Protein: 8g | Fat: 7g | Sugar: 1g

Variations and Tips

For diabetics: Reduce miso paste and soy sauce to lower sodium.
For allergies: Replace tofu with mushrooms for a soy-free option.
Flavor tip: Add fresh ginger or a dash of chili oil for a spicier version.

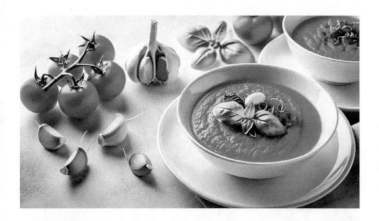

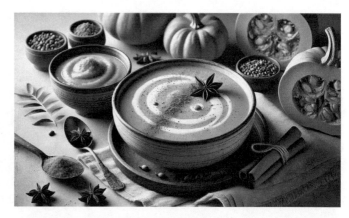

Roasted Tomato & Basil Soup with Garlic

Prep: 10 minutes   **Cook: 25 minutes**   **Serves: 2**

Ingredients:

- 500g tomatoes, halved
- 1 tbsp (15ml) olive oil
- 4 garlic cloves, unpeeled
- 1/2 onion (75g), diced
- 1/2 cup (120ml) vegetable broth
- 1 tbsp (10g) fresh basil, chopped
- Salt and pepper to taste

Instructions:

1. **Roast tomatoes and garlic**: Preheat oven to 200°C (400°F). Place tomatoes and garlic on a baking sheet, drizzle with olive oil, and roast for 20 minutes.
2. **Sauté onion**: In a pot, sauté onion in olive oil over medium heat for 5 minutes until softened.
3. **Blend**: Squeeze roasted garlic out of the skins and add to the pot along with the roasted tomatoes. Add broth, blend with an immersion blender until smooth.
4. **Finish and serve**: Stir in basil, season with salt and pepper, and serve hot.

Nutritional Facts (Per Serving):
Calories: 180 | Carbs: 20g | Protein: 4g | Fat: 10g | Sugar: 12g

Variations and Tips

For diabetics: Use fewer tomatoes or add zucchini to lower sugar content.
For allergies: Use bone broth instead of vegetable broth for added protein.
Flavor tip: Add a dash of balsamic vinegar for extra depth

Spiced Pumpkin Soup with Cumin & Coriander

Prep: 10 minutes   **Cook:20 minutes**   **Serves: 2**

Ingredients:

- 300g pumpkin, cubed
- 1 tbsp (15ml) olive oil
- 1/2 onion (75g), diced
- 1 garlic clove, minced
- 1/2 tsp (2g) ground cumin
- 1/2 tsp (2g) ground coriander
- 2 cups (480ml) vegetable broth
- 1 tbsp (15ml) coconut milk (optional)
- Salt and pepper to taste

Instructions:

1. **Sauté onion and garlic**: Heat olive oil in a pot over medium heat. Add onion and garlic, cook for 5 minutes until softened.
2. **Add pumpkin and spices**: Add pumpkin, cumin, and coriander. Cook for 3 minutes to release the flavors.
3. **Simmer**: Add broth, bring to a boil, then reduce heat and simmer for 15 minutes until pumpkin is tender.
4. **Blend and serve**: Blend the soup until smooth, stir in coconut milk (if using), and season to taste.

Nutritional Facts (Per Serving):
Calories: 200 | Carbs: 28g | Protein: 3g | Fat: 8g | Sugar: 10g

Variations and Tips

For diabetics: Replace some pumpkin with cauliflower for fewer carbs.
For allergies: Use almond milk instead of coconut milk for a nutty flavor.
Flavor tip: Add a pinch of chili powder for a spicier kick.

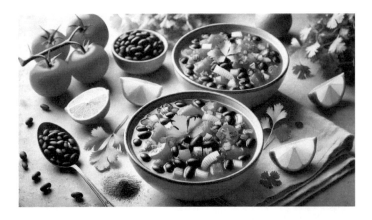

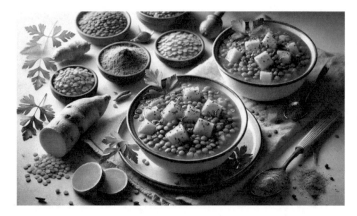

Zesty Lime & Black Bean Soup

Prep: 10 minutes   Cook: 20 minutes   Serves: 2

Ingredients:

- 1 can (400g) black beans, drained and rinsed
- 1 tbsp (15ml) olive oil
- 1/2 onion (75g), diced
- 1 garlic clove, minced
- 1/2 tsp (2g) ground cumin
- 1/2 tsp (2g) ground coriander
- 2 cups (480ml) vegetable broth
- 1/2 cup (120g) diced tomatoes
- 1 tbsp (15ml) lime juice
- Salt and pepper to taste
- Fresh cilantro for garnish

Instructions:

1. **Sauté onion and garlic**: Heat olive oil in a pot over medium heat. Add onion and garlic, cook for 5 minutes.
2. **Add spices and broth**: Stir in cumin and coriander. Add vegetable broth, black beans, and tomatoes. Simmer for 15 minutes.
3. **Finish with lime**: Stir in lime juice, season with salt and pepper. Serve garnished with fresh cilantro.

Nutritional Facts (Per Serving):
Calories: 280 | Carbs: 35g | Protein: 12g | Fat: 8g | Sugar: 4g

Variations and Tips

For diabetics: Use fewer tomatoes and add more vegetables like zucchini to lower sugar content.
For allergies: Replace black beans with chickpeas if sensitive to legumes.
Flavor tip: Add a pinch of smoked paprika for an extra layer of flavor

Lentil & Sweet Potato Soup

Prep: 10 minutes   Cook:25 minutes   Serves: 2

Ingredients:

- 1/2 cup (100g) red lentils
- 1 medium sweet potato (200g), diced
- 1 tbsp (15ml) olive oil
- 1/2 onion (75g), diced
- 1 garlic clove, minced
- 1 tsp (5g) ground turmeric
- 1/2 tsp (2g) ground cumin
- 3 cups (720ml) vegetable broth
- Salt and pepper to taste
- Fresh parsley for garnish

Instructions:

1. **Sauté onion and garlic**: Heat olive oil in a pot over medium heat. Add onion and garlic, cook for 5 minutes.
2. **Add sweet potato and spices**: Stir in sweet potato, turmeric, and cumin. Cook for 3 minutes.
3. **Simmer with lentils**: Add vegetable broth and lentils. Simmer for 20 minutes until lentils and sweet potato are tender.
4. **Serve**: Season with salt and pepper, garnish with fresh parsley.

Nutritional Facts (Per Serving):
Calories: 320 | Carbs: 50g | Protein: 12g | Fat: 8g | Sugar: 9g

Variations and Tips

For diabetics: Reduce sweet potato and add cauliflower for fewer carbs.
For allergies: Replace lentils with quinoa for a legume-free option.
Flavor tip: Add a squeeze of lemon for brightness and extra healing benefits.

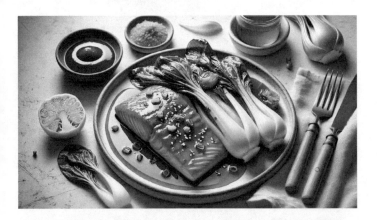

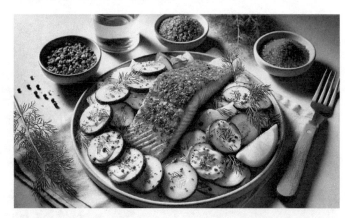

Miso Glazed Salmon with Bok Choy

Prep: 10 minutes   Cook: 15 minutes   Serves: 2

Ingredients:

- 2 salmon fillets (150g each)
- 1 tbsp (15ml) miso paste
- 1 tbsp (15ml) olive oil
- 1 tbsp (15ml) rice vinegar
- 1 tbsp (15ml) soy sauce (optional for extra flavor)
- 1 tbsp (15ml) honey
- 2 baby bok choy (200g), halved
- 1 garlic clove, minced
- Salt and pepper to taste

Instructions:

1. **Prepare the glaze**: In a bowl, mix miso paste, olive oil, rice vinegar, soy sauce (optional), and honey.
2. **Cook salmon**: Heat a skillet over medium heat. Sear salmon fillets skin-side down for 4-5 minutes. Brush miso glaze on top and continue cooking for another 5 minutes until salmon is cooked through.
3. **Sauté bok choy**: In a separate pan, sauté garlic in olive oil for 1 minute. Add bok choy, season with salt and pepper, and cook for 5 minutes until tender.
4. **Serve**: Plate the salmon with bok choy and drizzle with remaining glaze.

Nutritional Facts (Per Serving):
Calories: 350 | Carbs: 10g | Protein: 30g | Fat: 20g | Sugar: 7g

Variations and Tips

For diabetics: Reduce honey or omit for a lower sugar option.
For allergies: Use coconut aminos instead of soy sauce for a soy-free version.
Flavor tip: Add fresh ginger to the glaze for an extra zing.

Spiced Salmon with Cucumber Dill Salad

Prep: 10 minutes   Cook:10 minutes   Serves: 2

Ingredients:

- 2 salmon fillets (150g each)
- 1 tsp (5g) ground cumin
- 1/2 tsp (2g) ground paprika
- 1 tbsp (15ml) olive oil
- Salt and pepper to taste
- 1 cucumber (150g), thinly sliced
- 2 tbsp (30g) fresh dill, chopped
- 1 tbsp (15ml) lemon juice
- 1 tbsp (15ml) Greek yogurt (optional for creaminess)

Instructions:

1. **Season and cook salmon**: Rub salmon fillets with cumin, paprika, salt, and pepper. Heat olive oil in a pan over medium heat and cook salmon for 4-5 minutes on each side until cooked through.
2. **Prepare cucumber salad**: In a bowl, mix cucumber slices, dill, lemon juice, and Greek yogurt (if using). Toss to combine.
3. **Serve**: Plate the salmon with the cucumber dill salad on the side.

Nutritional Facts (Per Serving):
Calories: 300 | Carbs: 8g | Protein: 28g | Fat: 18g | Sugar: 2g

Variations and Tips

For diabetics: Omit yogurt or use a low-carb alternative.
For allergies: Replace Greek yogurt with a dairy-free option.
Flavor tip: Add a pinch of cayenne pepper to the salmon for a spicy kick

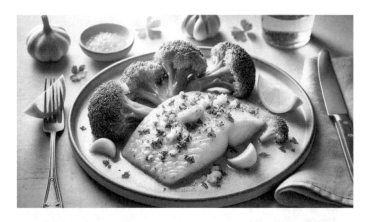

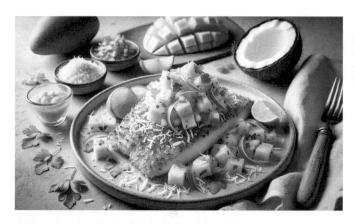

Garlic Butter Tilapia with Steamed Broccoli

Prep: 10 minutes   Cook: 15 minutes   Serves: 2

Ingredients:

- 2 tilapia fillets (150g each)
- 2 tbsp (30g) unsalted butter
- 2 garlic cloves, minced
- 1 tbsp (15ml) olive oil
- 1/2 lemon, juiced
- 200g broccoli florets
- Salt and pepper to taste
- Fresh parsley for garnish

Instructions:

1. **Steam the broccoli**: Steam the broccoli florets for 5-7 minutes until tender.
2. **Cook the tilapia**: In a skillet, heat olive oil over medium heat. Season tilapia with salt and pepper. Cook fillets for 3-4 minutes on each side until golden and cooked through.
3. **Make garlic butter**: In the same pan, melt the butter and add minced garlic. Cook for 1-2 minutes until fragrant. Squeeze lemon juice over the tilapia and drizzle garlic butter on top.
4. **Serve**: Plate the tilapia with steamed broccoli and garnish with fresh parsley.

Nutritional Facts (Per Serving):
Calories: 320 | Carbs: 6g | Protein: 28g | Fat: 21g | Sugar: 2g

Variations and Tips

For diabetics: Use less butter and olive oil to reduce fats.
For allergies: Replace butter with ghee or dairy-free alternatives.
Flavor tip: Add red pepper flakes to the garlic butter for a spicy kick

Coconut-Crusted Tilapia with Mango Salsa

Prep: 15 minutes   Cook: 10 minutes   Serves: 2

Ingredients:

- 2 tilapia fillets (150g each)
- 1/2 cup (50g) unsweetened shredded coconut
- 1/4 cup (30g) almond flour
- 1 egg, beaten
- 1 tbsp (15ml) coconut oil
- Salt and pepper to taste

Mango Salsa:

- 1 ripe mango, diced
- 1/4 cup (30g) red onion, diced
- 1 tbsp (15ml) lime juice
- 1 tbsp (10g) fresh cilantro, chopped
- Salt to taste

Instructions:

1. **Prepare the tilapia**: Season fillets with salt and pepper. Dip each fillet into the beaten egg, then coat with the mixture of shredded coconut and almond flour.
2. **Cook the tilapia**: Heat coconut oil in a pan over medium heat. Cook the tilapia for 3-4 minutes on each side until the coconut crust is golden brown and the fish is cooked through.
3. **Make the mango salsa**: In a bowl, mix the diced mango, red onion, lime juice, cilantro, and salt.
4. **Serve**: Plate the coconut-crusted tilapia and top with mango salsa

Nutritional Facts (Per Serving):
Calories: 400 | Carbs:20g | Protein:28g | Fat:22g | Sugar:10g

Variations and Tips

For diabetics: Reduce the amount of mango or replace with avocado for a lower sugar option.
For allergies: Replace almond flour with gluten-free flour or coconut flour.
Flavor tip: Add a pinch of cayenne to the coconut crust for a hint of heat

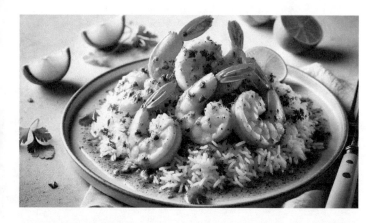

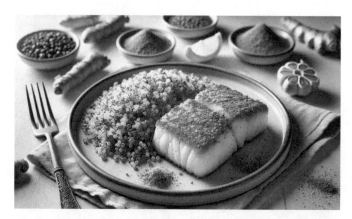

Coconut Lime Shrimp with Cilantro Rice

Prep: 10 minutes   Cook: 15 minutes   Serves: 2

Ingredients:

- 200g shrimp, peeled and deveined
- 1 tbsp (15ml) coconut oil
- 1/2 cup (120ml) coconut milk
- 1 tbsp (15ml) lime juice
- 1 garlic clove, minced
- 1/2 tsp (2g) ground cumin
- Salt and pepper to taste

Instructions:

1. **Cook the rice**: In a pot, combine basmati rice and water. Bring to a boil, then reduce heat to low, cover, and cook for 12-15 minutes. Once done, fluff with a fork and mix in chopped cilantro and lime juice.
2. **Sauté the shrimp**: Heat coconut oil in a pan over medium heat. Add shrimp and garlic, sauté for 3-4 minutes until shrimp turn pink.
3. **Make the sauce**: Stir in coconut milk, lime juice, cumin, salt, and pepper. Simmer for 2-3 minutes until the sauce thickens slightly.
4. **Serve**: Plate the shrimp over cilantro rice, drizzling the coconut lime sauce on top

Nutritional Facts (Per Serving):
Calories: 380 | Carbs: 30g | Protein: 20g | Fat: 18g | Sugar: 2g

Variations and Tips

For diabetics: Replace basmati rice with cauliflower rice for a lower carb option.
For allergies: Replace coconut milk with almond milk for a nutty flavor.
Flavor tip: Add red pepper flakes for a spicy kick

Turmeric-Crusted Cod with Quinoa

Prep: 10 minutes   Cook: 20 minutes   Serves: 2

Ingredients:

- 2 cod fillets (150g each)
- 1 tbsp (15ml) olive oil
- 1 tsp (5g) ground turmeric
- 1/2 tsp (2g) ground cumin
- Salt and pepper to taste
- 1/2 cup (90g) quinoa
- 1 cup (240ml) vegetable broth

Instructions:

1. **Cook the quinoa**: In a pot, bring vegetable broth to a boil. Add quinoa, reduce heat, cover, and simmer for 15 minutes until all liquid is absorbed.
2. **Season the cod**: Mix turmeric, cumin, salt, and pepper. Rub the spice mixture onto both sides of the cod fillets.
3. **Cook the cod**: Heat olive oil in a pan over medium heat. Sear cod fillets for 3-4 minutes on each side until golden and cooked through.
4. **Serve**: Plate the turmeric-crusted cod with quinoa on the side

Nutritional Facts (Per Serving):
Calories: 350 | Carbs: 30g | Protein:28g | Fat:12g | Sugar: 1g

Variations and Tips

For diabetics: Replace quinoa with zucchini noodles or another low-carb vegetable.
For allergies: Use cauliflower rice instead of quinoa for a grain-free option.
Flavor tip: Add a squeeze of lemon for a bright finish

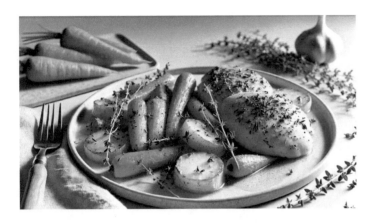

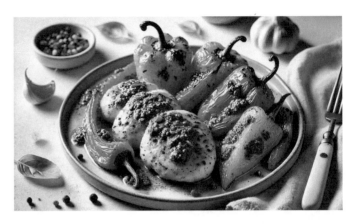

Thyme-Roasted Chicken with Carrots and Parsnips

Prep: 10 minutes   Cook: 35 minutes   Serves: 2

Ingredients:

- 2 chicken breasts (200g each)
- 2 tbsp (30ml) olive oil
- 1 tbsp (15g) fresh thyme leaves
- 2 carrots (150g), peeled and chopped
- 2 parsnips (150g), peeled and chopped
- 2 garlic cloves, minced
- Salt and pepper to taste

Instructions:

1. **Preheat the oven**: Preheat the oven to 200°C (400°F).
2. **Prepare vegetables**: Toss the carrots, parsnips, and garlic with 1 tbsp olive oil, salt, pepper, and half of the thyme. Spread evenly on a baking sheet.
3. **Season the chicken**: Rub the chicken breasts with the remaining olive oil, thyme, salt, and pepper. Place them on top of the vegetables.
4. **Roast**: Roast in the oven for 30-35 minutes, until the chicken is cooked through and the vegetables are tender.
5. **Serve**: Slice the chicken and serve it with the roasted vegetables.

Nutritional Facts (Per Serving):
Calories: 450 | Carbs: 20g | Protein: 35g | Fat: 25g | Sugar: 8g

Variations and Tips

For diabetics: Replace parsnips with more carrots or zucchini to lower the carb content.
For allergies: Replace chicken with tofu for a vegetarian option.
Flavor tip: Add a squeeze of lemon juice over the chicken for a fresh twist.

Pesto Chicken with Roasted Bell Peppers

Prep: 10 minutes   Cook: 25 minutes   Serves: 2

Ingredients:

- 2 chicken breasts (200g each)
- 1/4 cup (60g) pesto (homemade or store-bought)
- 1 tbsp (15ml) olive oil
- 2 bell peppers (200g), sliced
- Salt and pepper to taste

Instructions:

1. **Preheat the oven**: Preheat the oven to 200°C (400°F).
2. **Prepare the bell peppers**: Toss the sliced bell peppers with olive oil, salt, and pepper. Spread them on a baking sheet.
3. **Season the chicken**: Rub the chicken breasts with pesto, then place them on the baking sheet with the bell peppers.
4. **Roast**: Bake for 25 minutes until the chicken is cooked through and the peppers are soft and slightly caramelized.
5. **Serve**: Slice the chicken and serve it with the roasted bell peppers.

Nutritional Facts (Per Serving):
Calories: 400 | Carbs: 12g | Protein:35g | Fat:22g | Sugar: 6g

Variations and Tips

For diabetics: Use a low-carb pesto or make your own with extra greens like spinach.
For allergies: Replace pesto with a dairy-free version if needed.
Flavor tip: Garnish with extra fresh basil or pine nuts for added crunch.

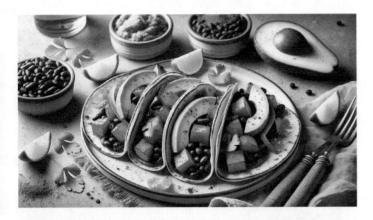

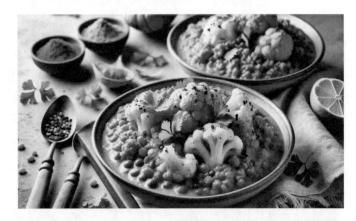

Sweet Potato & Black Bean Tacos with Avocado

Prep: 10 minutes   Cook: 20 minutes   Serves: 2

Ingredients:

- 1 medium sweet potato (200g), peeled and diced
- 1 tbsp (15ml) olive oil
- 1/2 cup (120g) black beans, cooked
- 1/2 tsp (2g) ground cumin
- 1/2 tsp (2g) smoked paprika
- Salt and pepper to taste
- 4 small corn tortillas
- 1 avocado, sliced
- Fresh cilantro for garnish
- 1 lime, sliced

Instructions:

1. **Roast sweet potatoes**: Preheat oven to 200°C (400°F). Toss diced sweet potatoes with olive oil, cumin, smoked paprika, salt, and pepper. Spread on a baking sheet and roast for 15-20 minutes until tender.
2. **Heat black beans**: In a pan, warm the cooked black beans over medium heat, adding a pinch of salt and pepper.
3. **Assemble tacos**: Warm tortillas, then fill with roasted sweet potatoes, black beans, and avocado slices. Garnish with fresh cilantro and a squeeze of lime.
4. **Serve**: Serve immediately with extra lime wedges on the side

Nutritional Facts (Per Serving):
Calories: 350 | Carbs: 50g | Protein: 9g | Fat: 15g | Sugar: 5g

Variations and Tips

For diabetics: Use low-carb tortillas or lettuce wraps instead of corn tortillas.
For allergies: Use gluten-free tortillas if needed.
Flavor tip: Add a dash of hot sauce or pickled jalapeños for extra spice

Coconut Curry Lentil Stew with Cauliflower

Prep: 10 minutes   Cook:30 minutes   Serves: 2

Ingredients:

- 1/2 cup (100g) red lentils
- 1/2 head of cauliflower (200g), cut into florets
- 1 tbsp (15ml) coconut oil
- 1 garlic clove, minced
- 1 tbsp (15g) curry powder
- 1/2 tsp (2g) ground turmeric
- 1 can (400ml) coconut milk
- 1 cup (240ml) vegetable broth
- Salt and pepper to taste
- Fresh cilantro for garnish

Instructions:

1. **Sauté garlic and spices**: In a large pot, heat coconut oil over medium heat. Add minced garlic, curry powder, and turmeric. Cook for 1-2 minutes until fragrant.
2. **Add lentils and broth**: Stir in red lentils and vegetable broth. Bring to a boil, then reduce heat and simmer for 10 minutes.
3. **Add coconut milk and cauliflower**: Stir in coconut milk and cauliflower florets. Simmer for another 15 minutes until the lentils and cauliflower are tender.
4. **Serve**: Season with salt and pepper, and garnish with fresh cilantro before serving

Nutritional Facts (Per Serving):
Calories: 400 | Carbs: 35g | Protein:12g | Fat:25g | Sugar: 4g

Variations and Tips

For diabetics: Reduce coconut milk or use a light version to lower fat content.
For allergies: Replace coconut milk with almond milk or another dairy-free option.
Flavor tip: Add a squeeze of lemon juice for brightness and extra anti-inflammatory benefits.

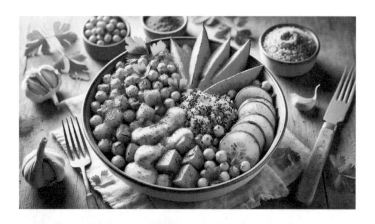

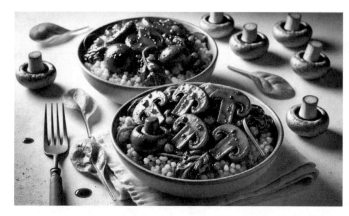

Chickpea & Sweet Potato Bowl with Garlic Tahini

Prep: 10 minutes   Cook: 25 minutes   Serves: 2

Ingredients:

- 1 medium sweet potato (200g), peeled and diced
- 1 tbsp (15ml) olive oil
- 1/2 cup (120g) cooked chickpeas
- 1/2 tsp (2g) ground cumin
- 1/2 tsp (2g) smoked paprika
- Salt and pepper to taste
- 1/2 cup (120g) quinoa, cooked
- 1/4 cup (60g) cucumber, diced
- Fresh parsley for garnish

Garlic Tahini Dressing:

- 2 tbsp (30g) tahini
- 1 garlic clove, minced
- 1 tbsp (15ml) lemon juice
- 2 tbsp (30ml) water
- Salt to taste

Instructions:

1. **Roast the sweet potatoes**: Preheat oven to 200°C (400°F). Toss diced sweet potatoes with olive oil, cumin, smoked paprika, salt, and pepper. Spread on a baking sheet and roast for 20-25 minutes until tender.
2. **Prepare chickpeas**: Warm cooked chickpeas in a pan with a pinch of salt and pepper for 2-3 minutes.
3. **Make the garlic tahini dressing**: In a small bowl, whisk together tahini, garlic, lemon juice, water, and salt until smooth.
4. **Assemble the bowl**: Divide the quinoa between two bowls. Top with roasted sweet potatoes, chickpeas, cucumber, and drizzle with garlic tahini dressing. Garnish with fresh parsley

Nutritional Facts (Per Serving):
Calories: 400 | Carbs: 50g | Protein: 12g | Fat: 16g | Sugar: 4g

Variations and Tips

For diabetics: Use cauliflower rice instead of quinoa for a lower carb option.
For allergies: Replace tahini with almond or sunflower seed butter for a nut-free version.
Flavor tip: Add roasted red peppers or pickled onions for extra flavor and texture.

Balsamic Glazed Mushroom & Farro Stir Fry

Prep: 10 minutes   Cook: 20 minutes   Serves: 2

Ingredients:

- 1 cup (100g) mushrooms, sliced
- 1/2 cup (90g) farro, cooked
- 1 tbsp (15ml) olive oil
- 2 tbsp (30ml) balsamic vinegar
- 1 garlic clove, minced
- 1/4 tsp (1g) crushed red pepper flakes (optional)
- 1/2 cup (60g) spinach
- Salt and pepper to taste

Instructions:

1. **Cook mushrooms**: Heat olive oil in a large pan over medium heat. Add sliced mushrooms and sauté for 5-7 minutes until browned.
2. **Add garlic and balsamic**: Stir in minced garlic, balsamic vinegar, and crushed red pepper flakes (if using). Cook for another 2-3 minutes until the mushrooms are well-coated and the balsamic slightly reduces.
3. **Stir in spinach and farro**: Add cooked farro and spinach to the pan. Stir and cook for 3-4 minutes until the spinach wilts and everything is heated through.
4. **Serve**: Season with salt and pepper and serve immediately.

Nutritional Facts (Per Serving):
Calories: 350 | Carbs: 45g | Protein:10g | Fat:12g | Sugar: 6g

Variations and Tips

For diabetics: Use quinoa or cauliflower rice in place of farro for a lower carb option.
For allergies: Omit crushed red pepper flakes if sensitive to spice.
Flavor tip: Garnish with fresh basil or pine nuts for an extra layer of flavor and texture

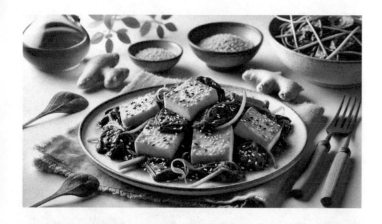

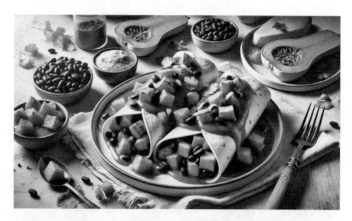

Crispy Tofu with Ginger Sesame Spinach

Prep: 10 minutes   Cook: 20 minutes   Serves: 2

Ingredients:

- 200g firm tofu, pressed and cubed
- 1 tbsp (15ml) sesame oil
- 1 tbsp (15ml) tamari or soy sauce
- 1 tsp (5g) fresh ginger, minced
- 2 cups (60g) fresh spinach
- 1 tsp (5g) sesame seeds
- 1 garlic clove, minced
- Salt and pepper to taste

Instructions:

1. **Prepare the tofu**: Press tofu to remove excess moisture, then cube it. In a pan, heat sesame oil over medium heat. Add tofu cubes and cook for 5-7 minutes, turning occasionally, until golden and crispy.
2. **Cook the spinach**: In the same pan, after tofu is cooked, add minced garlic and ginger. Sauté for 1 minute. Add fresh spinach and cook until wilted, about 2-3 minutes.
3. **Season and garnish**: Drizzle with tamari or soy sauce and sprinkle sesame seeds on top. Serve tofu over the sautéed spinach.

Nutritional Facts (Per Serving):
Calories: 280 | Carbs: 8g | Protein: 16g | Fat: 20g | Sugar: 1g

Variations and Tips

For diabetics: Use reduced-sodium tamari or soy sauce to control salt intake.
For allergies: Use coconut aminos instead of soy sauce for a soy-free option.
Flavor tip: Add a splash of rice vinegar or lime juice for a tangy kick.

Butternut Squash and Black Bean Enchiladas

Prep: 15 minutes   Cook: 30 minutes   Serves: 2

Ingredients:

- 1 cup (150g) butternut squash, peeled and diced
- 1/2 cup (120g) black beans, cooked
- 4 small corn tortillas
- 1/2 cup (120ml) enchilada sauce (homemade or store-bought)
- 1 tbsp (15ml) olive oil
- 1/2 tsp (2g) cumin
- 1/2 tsp (2g) smoked paprika
- Salt and pepper to taste
- Fresh cilantro for garnish

Instructions:

1. **Roast the butternut squash**: Preheat oven to 200°C (400°F). Toss the diced butternut squash with olive oil, cumin, smoked paprika, salt, and pepper. Spread on a baking sheet and roast for 20-25 minutes until tender.
2. **Assemble the enchiladas**: Warm the tortillas, then fill each one with roasted butternut squash and black beans. Roll them up and place them seam-side down in a baking dish.
3. **Bake**: Pour the enchilada sauce over the rolled tortillas. Bake for 10 minutes until heated through.
4. **Serve**: Garnish with fresh cilantro before serving

Nutritional Facts (Per Serving):
Calories: 350 | Carbs: 50g | Protein:10g | Fat:12g | Sugar: 6g

Variations and Tips

For diabetics: Use low-carb tortillas or lettuce wraps to reduce carbohydrate content.
For allergies: Substitute corn tortillas with gluten-free tortillas if necessary.
Flavor tip: Add avocado slices on top for creaminess and extra healthy fats.

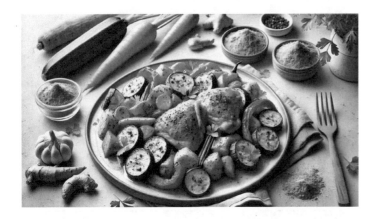

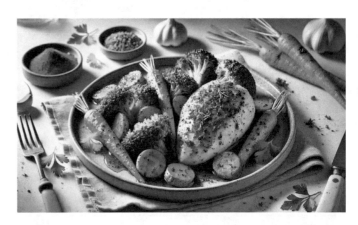

Turmeric-Roasted Vegetables with Chicken Thighs

Prep: 10 minutes   Cook: 35 minutes   Serves: 2

Ingredients:

- 4 chicken thighs (about 400g)
- 1 tbsp (15ml) olive oil
- 1 tsp (5g) ground turmeric
- 1/2 tsp (2g) cumin
- 1/2 tsp (2g) smoked paprika
- 1 sweet potato (200g), peeled and diced
- 1 red bell pepper (150g), sliced
- 1 zucchini (150g), sliced
- Salt and pepper to taste
- Fresh parsley for garnish

Instructions:

1. **Preheat the oven**: Preheat oven to 200°C (400°F).
2. **Prepare the vegetables**: Toss the sweet potato, bell pepper, and zucchini with olive oil, turmeric, cumin, smoked paprika, salt, and pepper. Spread evenly on a baking sheet.
3. **Season the chicken**: Rub the chicken thighs with olive oil, salt, and pepper. Place them on the baking sheet with the vegetables.
4. **Roast**: Roast for 30-35 minutes, until the chicken thighs are golden and cooked through, and the vegetables are tender.
5. **Serve**: Garnish with fresh parsley and serve immediately.

Nutritional Facts (Per Serving):
Calories: 450 | Carbs: 25g | Protein: 35g | Fat: 22g | Sugar: 6g

Variations and Tips

For diabetics: Replace the sweet potato with cauliflower or more zucchini to reduce carbs.
For allergies: Substitute chicken thighs with tofu or tempeh for a plant-based option.
Flavor tip: Add a squeeze of lemon juice before serving for added brightness.

Paprika Chicken with Roasted Broccoli and Carrots

Prep: 10 minutes   Cook:30 minutes   Serves: 2

Ingredients:

- 4 chicken thighs (about 400g)
- 1 tbsp (15ml) olive oil
- 1 tsp (5g) ground turmeric
- 1/2 tsp (2g) cumin
- 1/2 tsp (2g) smoked paprika
- 1 sweet potato (200g), peeled and diced
- 1 red bell pepper (150g), sliced
- 1 zucchini (150g), sliced
- Salt and pepper to taste
- Fresh parsley for garnish

Instructions:

1. **Preheat the oven**: Preheat oven to 200°C (400°F).
2. **Prepare the vegetables**: Toss the sweet potato, bell pepper, and zucchini with olive oil, turmeric, cumin, smoked paprika, salt, and pepper. Spread evenly on a baking sheet.
3. **Season the chicken**: Rub the chicken thighs with olive oil, salt, and pepper. Place them on the baking sheet with the vegetables.
4. **Roast**: Roast for 30-35 minutes, until the chicken thighs are golden and cooked through, and the vegetables are tender.
5. **Serve**: Garnish with fresh parsley and serve immediately.

Nutritional Facts (Per Serving):
Calories: 450 | Carbs: 25g | Protein:35g | Fat:22g | Sugar: 6g

Variations and Tips

For diabetics: Replace the sweet potato with cauliflower or more zucchini to reduce carbs.
For allergies: Substitute chicken thighs with tofu or tempeh for a plant-based option.
Flavor tip: Add a squeeze of lemon juice before serving for added brightness.

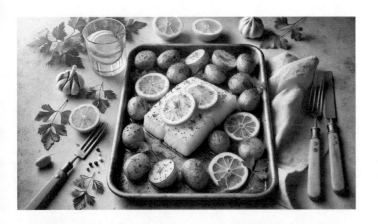

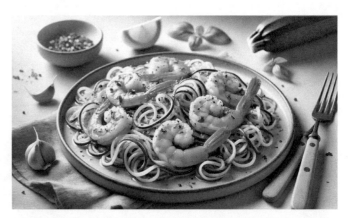

Sheet Pan Cod with Lemon and Dill Potatoes

Prep: 10 minutes   Cook: 25 minutes   Serves: 2

Ingredients:

- 2 cod fillets (about 300g)
- 200g baby potatoes, halved
- 1 tbsp (15ml) olive oil
- 1 lemon, sliced
- 2 tbsp fresh dill, chopped
- 1 garlic clove, minced
- Salt and pepper to taste
- Fresh parsley for garnish

Instructions:

1. **Preheat the oven**: Preheat oven to 200°C (400°F).
2. **Prepare the potatoes**: Toss the halved baby potatoes with olive oil, garlic, salt, and pepper. Spread them on a sheet pan and roast for 15 minutes.
3. **Add the cod**: After 15 minutes, push the potatoes to the side and place the cod fillets on the sheet pan. Top with lemon slices and sprinkle fresh dill on both the fish and potatoes. Roast for an additional 10 minutes or until the cod is cooked through and flakes easily with a fork.
4. **Serve**: Garnish with fresh parsley before serving

Nutritional Facts (Per Serving):
Calories: 350 | Carbs: 30g | Protein: 25g | Fat: 12g | Sugar: 2g

Variations and Tips

For diabetics: Replace the baby potatoes with cauliflower or zucchini for a lower-carb option.
For allergies: Substitute cod with tofu for a plant-based option.
Flavor tip: Add capers for a briny twist, or drizzle with extra lemon juice before serving.

One-Pan Garlic Shrimp with Zucchini Noodles

Prep: 10 minutes   Cook: 10 minutes   Serves: 2

Ingredients:

- 200g shrimp, peeled and deveined
- 2 medium zucchinis, spiralized into noodles
- 2 tbsp (30ml) olive oil
- 3 garlic cloves, minced
- 1/2 tsp red pepper flakes (optional)
- Juice of 1 lemon
- Salt and pepper to taste
- Fresh basil or parsley for garnish

Instructions:

1. **Cook the shrimp**: Heat 1 tbsp of olive oil in a large pan over medium heat. Add the shrimp, garlic, and red pepper flakes (if using). Cook for 3-4 minutes until shrimp are pink and cooked through. Remove shrimp from the pan and set aside.
2. **Cook the zucchini noodles**: In the same pan, add another tablespoon of olive oil. Toss in the zucchini noodles and sauté for 2-3 minutes until just tender.
3. **Combine and serve**: Return the shrimp to the pan with the zucchini noodles. Add lemon juice, salt, and pepper, and toss everything together. Garnish with fresh basil or parsley before serving

Nutritional Facts (Per Serving):
Calories: 300 | Carbs: 10g | Protein:25g | Fat:18g | Sugar: 3g

Variations and Tips

For diabetics: The dish is naturally low in carbs, but you can swap zucchini noodles for shirataki noodles for even fewer carbs.
For allergies: Replace shrimp with tempeh or tofu for a vegetarian option.
Flavor tip: Add a dash of white wine to the pan for extra flavor while cooking the shrimp.

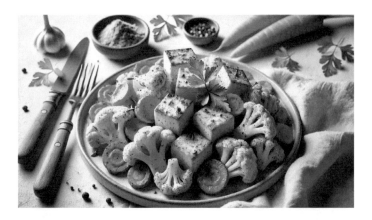 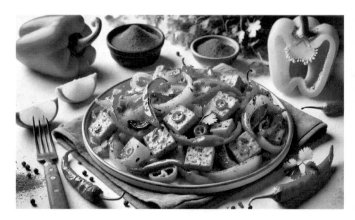

Crispy Tofu with Roasted Cauliflower and Carrots

Prep: 10 minutes   Cook: 25 minutes   Serves: 2

Ingredients:

- 200g firm tofu, pressed and cubed
- 1 tbsp (15ml) olive oil
- 1 tsp ground turmeric
- 1/2 tsp cumin
- 1/2 tsp smoked paprika
- 200g cauliflower florets
- 2 medium carrots (150g), sliced
- Salt and pepper to taste
- Fresh parsley for garnish

Instructions:

1. **Preheat the oven**: Preheat oven to 200°C (400°F).
2. **Prepare the vegetables**: Toss cauliflower florets and sliced carrots with 1/2 tbsp of olive oil, turmeric, cumin, smoked paprika, salt, and pepper. Spread on a baking sheet and roast for 25-30 minutes until tender.
3. **Cook the tofu**: While the vegetables roast, heat the remaining olive oil in a skillet over medium heat. Add the cubed tofu and cook for 5-7 minutes, turning occasionally, until golden and crispy on all sides.
4. **Serve**: Plate the crispy tofu with the roasted vegetables and garnish with fresh parsley.

Nutritional Facts (Per Serving):
Calories: 320 | Carbs: 25g | Protein: 15g | Fat: 18g | Sugar: 5g

Variations and Tips

For diabetics: Replace the carrots with zucchini or green beans to lower the carb content.
For allergies: Replace tofu with tempeh for a soy-free alternative.
Flavor tip: Add a drizzle of tahini or lemon juice before serving for extra depth

One-Pan Spicy Tempeh with Bell Peppers

Prep: 10 minutes   Cook: 15 minutes   Serves: 2

Ingredients:

- 200g tempeh, sliced
- 1 tbsp (15ml) olive oil
- 1 red bell pepper (150g), sliced
- 1 yellow bell pepper (150g), sliced
- 2 garlic cloves, minced
- 1 tsp chili powder
- 1/2 tsp smoked paprika
- Juice of 1 lime
- Salt and pepper to taste
- Fresh cilantro for garnish

Instructions:

1. **Cook the tempeh**: Heat olive oil in a large skillet over medium heat. Add sliced tempeh and cook for 5-7 minutes, turning until golden and slightly crispy.
2. **Add the vegetables**: Add the sliced bell peppers, garlic, chili powder, smoked paprika, salt, and pepper. Cook for 5-7 minutes until the peppers are softened.
3. **Finish and serve**: Squeeze lime juice over the dish and garnish with fresh cilantro before serving

Nutritional Facts (Per Serving):
Calories: 350 | Carbs: 20g | Protein:18g | Fat:20g | Sugar: 5g

Variations and Tips

For diabetics: Replace bell peppers with zucchini or green beans for a lower-carb option.
For allergies: Swap tempeh for seitan or mushrooms if allergic to soy.
Flavor tip: Add avocado slices or hot sauce for an extra kick of flavor.

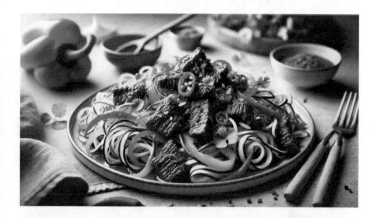

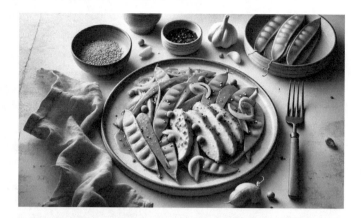

Spicy Beef Stir Fry with Zucchini Noodles

Prep: 10 minutes   **Cook: 15 minutes**   **Serves: 2**

Ingredients:

- 200g lean beef strips
- 2 medium zucchinis, spiralized into noodles
- 1 tbsp (15ml) olive oil
- 2 garlic cloves, minced
- 1 tsp chili flakes (adjust to taste)
- 1 tbsp (15ml) tamari (or soy sauce, gluten-free if needed)
- 1 tsp fresh ginger, minced
- 1/2 red bell pepper (75g), sliced
- 1/2 yellow bell pepper (75g), sliced
- Salt and pepper to taste
- Fresh cilantro for garnish

Instructions:

1. **Cook the beef**: Heat olive oil in a large pan over medium heat. Add the beef strips, garlic, and chili flakes. Stir-fry for 4-5 minutes until the beef is browned and cooked through.
2. **Add the vegetables**: Add the bell peppers and ginger to the pan. Stir-fry for 3-4 minutes until slightly softened.
3. **Cook the zucchini noodles**: In the same pan, add the zucchini noodles and tamari. Stir-fry for 2-3 minutes until just tender.
4. **Serve**: Garnish with fresh cilantro and serve immediately.

Nutritional Facts (Per Serving):
Calories: 350 | Carbs: 12g | Protein: 28g | Fat: 20g | Sugar: 4g

Variations and Tips

For diabetics: The dish is naturally low in carbs, but you can reduce tamari or soy sauce for less sodium.

For allergies: Replace beef with tofu or tempeh for a plant-based option.

Flavor tip: Add a dash of lime juice for extra zing before serving.

Ginger-Garlic Chicken Stir Fry with Snow Peas

Prep: 10 minutes   **Cook:15 minutes**   **Serves: 2**

Ingredients:

- 200g chicken breast, sliced into thin strips
- 1 tbsp (15ml) olive oil
- 2 garlic cloves, minced
- 1 tbsp (15ml) tamari (or soy sauce, gluten-free if needed)
- 1 tsp fresh ginger, minced
- 1 cup (100g) snow peas
- 1/2 cup (50g) sliced carrots
- 1 tbsp (15ml) sesame oil (optional)
- Salt and pepper to taste
- Fresh sesame seeds for garnish

Instructions:

1. **Preheat the oven**: Preheat oven to 200°C (400°F).
2. **Prepare the vegetables**: Toss the sweet potato, bell pepper, and zucchini with olive oil, turmeric, cumin, smoked paprika, salt, and pepper. Spread evenly on a baking sheet.
3. **Season the chicken**: Rub the chicken thighs with olive oil, salt, and pepper. Place them on the baking sheet with the vegetables.
4. **Roast**: Roast for 30-35 minutes, until the chicken thighs are golden and cooked through, and the vegetables are tender.
5. **Serve**: Garnish with fresh parsley and serve immediately.

Nutritional Facts (Per Serving):
Calories: 320 | Carbs: 10g | Protein:30g | Fat:18g | Sugar: 3g

Variations and Tips

For diabetics: Opt for low-sodium tamari or reduce the amount of tamari used.

For allergies: Replace chicken with tofu for a vegetarian option.

Flavor tip: Add a squeeze of lemon juice and a sprinkle of chili flakes for added brightness and heat.

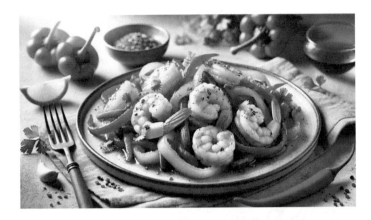

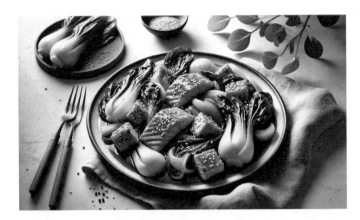

Spicy Shrimp Stir Fry with Bell Peppers

Prep: 10 minutes   Cook: 10 minutes   Serves: 2

Ingredients:

- 200g shrimp, peeled and deveined
- 1 tbsp (15ml) olive oil
- 1 red bell pepper (150g), sliced
- 1 yellow bell pepper (150g), sliced
- 2 garlic cloves, minced
- 1 tsp chili flakes (adjust to taste)
- 1 tbsp (15ml) tamari (or soy sauce, gluten-free if needed)
- 1 tsp fresh ginger, minced
- Salt and pepper to taste
- Fresh cilantro for garnish

Instructions:

1. **Cook the shrimp**: Heat olive oil in a large pan over medium heat. Add shrimp, garlic, and chili flakes. Stir-fry for 3-4 minutes until the shrimp turns pink and cooked through.
2. **Add the bell peppers**: Add sliced bell peppers and ginger. Stir-fry for another 3-4 minutes until the peppers are tender.
3. **Finish and serve**: Add tamari, season with salt and pepper, and stir well. Garnish with fresh cilantro before serving.

Nutritional Facts (Per Serving):
Calories: 250 | Carbs: 10g | Protein: 25g | Fat: 12g | Sugar: 4g

Variations and Tips

For diabetics: Use less tamari or choose a low-sodium version.
For allergies: Replace shrimp with tofu for a vegetarian option.
Flavor tip: Add a squeeze of lime juice for extra brightness.

Teriyaki Salmon Stir Fry with Bok Choy

Prep: 10 minutes   Cook: 12 minutes   Serves: 2

Ingredients:

- 200g salmon fillets, skin removed and cubed
- 1 tbsp (15ml) olive oil
- 2 cups (150g) bok choy, chopped
- 1 tbsp (15ml) homemade or store-bought teriyaki sauce (low-sodium)
- 1 garlic clove, minced
- 1 tsp fresh ginger, minced
- 1/4 cup (60ml) water
- 1 tbsp sesame oil (optional)
- Salt and pepper to taste
- Sesame seeds for garnish

Instructions:

1. **Cook the salmon**: Heat olive oil in a large pan over medium heat. Add salmon cubes and cook for 3-4 minutes, turning until browned on all sides.
2. **Add the bok choy**: Add garlic, ginger, and bok choy to the pan. Stir-fry for 3-4 minutes until bok choy softens slightly.
3. **Finish with teriyaki**: Add water and teriyaki sauce. Stir well and cook for another 2-3 minutes until the sauce thickens. Drizzle with sesame oil if using.
4. **Serve**: Garnish with sesame seeds before serving

Nutritional Facts (Per Serving):
Calories: 320 | Carbs: 12g | Protein:28g | Fat:18g | Sugar: 4g

Variations and Tips

For diabetics: Opt for a low-sugar teriyaki sauce or make your own with natural sweeteners.
For allergies: Replace salmon with tempeh or mushrooms for a vegetarian alternative.
Flavor tip: Add thinly sliced green onions for a fresh finish.

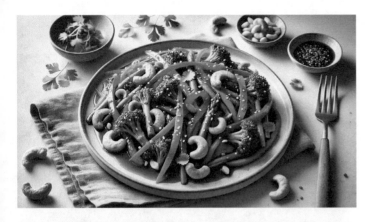

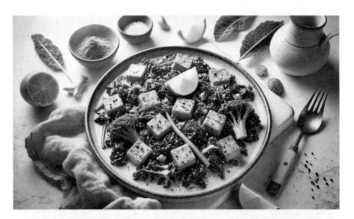

Miso Veggie Stir Fry with Cashews

Prep: 10 minutes   **Cook: 15 minutes**   **Serves: 2**

Ingredients:

- 1 tbsp (15ml) olive oil
- 1 medium carrot, sliced (100g)
- 1 red bell pepper, sliced (150g)
- 1 cup (100g) broccoli florets
- 1 tbsp (15ml) miso paste
- 1 tsp fresh ginger, minced
- 1 garlic clove, minced
- 2 tbsp (30ml) tamari (or soy sauce, gluten-free if needed)
- 1/4 cup (30g) unsalted cashews, toasted
- 1 tbsp sesame oil (optional)
- Salt and pepper to taste
- Fresh cilantro or green onions for garnish

Instructions:

4. **Heat the oil**: In a large pan, heat olive oil over medium heat.
5. **Cook the vegetables**: Add carrots, bell pepper, and broccoli. Stir-fry for 5-7 minutes until vegetables are tender but still crisp.
6. **Add flavor**: Stir in miso paste, ginger, garlic, and tamari. Cook for another 2-3 minutes to combine flavors.
7. **Finish and serve**: Add toasted cashews and sesame oil if using. Stir well and garnish with fresh cilantro or green onions before serving.

Nutritional Facts (Per Serving):
Calories: 280 | Carbs: 22g | Protein: 8g | Fat: 18g | Sugar: 5g

Variations and Tips

For diabetics: Substitute carrots with zucchini or more broccoli for a lower-carb option.
For allergies: Replace cashews with sunflower seeds for a nut-free version.
Flavor tip: Add a dash of lime juice for extra brightness before serving.

Coconut Ginger Tofu Stir Fry with Kale

Prep: 10 minutes   **Cook: 15 minutes**   **Serves: 2**

Ingredients:

- 200g firm tofu, pressed and cubed
- 1 tbsp (15ml) coconut oil
- 2 garlic cloves, minced
- 1 tsp fresh ginger, minced
- 2 cups (150g) kale, chopped
- 1/2 cup (120ml) coconut milk (full-fat)
- 1 tbsp (15ml) tamari (or soy sauce, gluten-free if needed)
- 1/2 tsp turmeric powder
- 1/4 tsp red pepper flakes (optional)
- Salt and pepper to taste
- Fresh lime wedges for garnish

Instructions:

5. **Cook the tofu**: Heat coconut oil in a large pan over medium heat. Add cubed tofu and cook for 5-7 minutes, turning until golden and crispy.
6. **Add the garlic and ginger**: Add minced garlic and ginger to the pan and stir for 1-2 minutes until fragrant.
7. **Add the kale**: Stir in chopped kale, coconut milk, tamari, turmeric, and red pepper flakes (if using). Cook for another 3-4 minutes until kale is wilted and flavors are combined.
8. **Serve**: Season with salt and pepper, then garnish with fresh lime wedges before serving.

Nutritional Facts (Per Serving):
Calories: 320 | Carbs: 10g | Protein:14g | Fat:26g | Sugar: 2g

Variations and Tips

For diabetics: Reduce the amount of coconut milk or replace it with almond milk for a lower-fat version.
For allergies: Use sunflower seed oil instead of coconut oil if allergic to coconut.
Flavor tip: Sprinkle with toasted sesame seeds for added crunch and flavor.

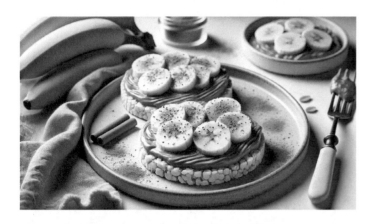

Peanut Butter Banana Rice Cakes

Prep: 5 minutes   **Cook: N/A**   **Serves: 2**

Ingredients:

- 2 rice cakes
- 2 tbsp (30g) natural peanut butter (without added sugar)
- 1 medium banana, sliced (100g)
- 1/2 tsp cinnamon (optional)
- 1 tsp chia seeds (optional)

Instructions:

1. **Assemble the rice cakes**: Spread 1 tbsp of peanut butter on each rice cake.
2. **Add the toppings**: Arrange banana slices on top of the peanut butter.
3. **Optional garnish**: Sprinkle with cinnamon and chia seeds for added flavor and texture.
4. **Serve**: Enjoy immediately as a quick snack or breakfast.

Nutritional Facts (Per Serving):
Calories: 220 | Carbs: 30g | Protein: 7g | Fat: 9g | Sugar: 9g

Variations and Tips

For diabetics: Use almond butter instead of peanut butter to reduce sugar content.
For allergies: Replace peanut butter with sunflower seed butter for a nut-free option.
Flavor tip: Add a drizzle of honey or maple syrup for extra sweetness.

Roasted Beet Chips with Sea Salt

Prep: 10 minutes   **Cook: 30 minutes**   **Serves: 2**

Ingredients:

- 2 medium beets (200g), thinly sliced
- 1 tbsp (15ml) olive oil
- 1/2 tsp sea salt
- 1/4 tsp black pepper (optional)

Instructions:

1. **Preheat the oven**: Preheat your oven to 180°C (350°F).
2. **Prepare the beets**: Thinly slice the beets using a mandoline or knife. Toss them with olive oil, sea salt, and black pepper.
3. **Roast the chips**: Lay the beet slices in a single layer on a baking sheet. Roast for 25-30 minutes, flipping halfway through, until crispy.
4. **Serve**: Let the beet chips cool for a few minutes before serving.

Nutritional Facts (Per Serving):
Calories: 110 | Carbs: 15g | Protein: 2g | Fat: 5g | Sugar: 9g

Variations and Tips

For diabetics: Use golden beets, which are lower in sugar than red beets.
For allergies: The recipe is naturally allergen-free, but you can use avocado oil instead of olive oil for variation.
Flavor tip: Sprinkle with a pinch of smoked paprika or rosemary for extra flavor

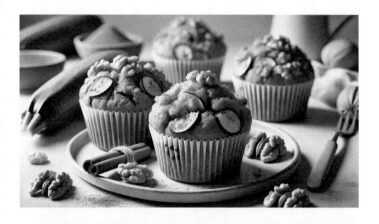

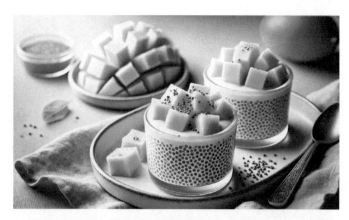

Zucchini Muffins with Walnuts and Cinnamon

Prep: 10 minutes   Cook: 20 minutes   Serves: 2

Ingredients:

- 1 cup (125g) grated zucchini
- 1/2 cup (60g) almond flour
- 1/4 cup (30g) walnuts, chopped
- 1 large egg
- 1 tbsp (15ml) olive oil
- 2 tbsp (30ml) maple syrup
- 1 tsp cinnamon
- 1/2 tsp baking powder
- 1/4 tsp sea salt

Instructions:

1. **Preheat the oven**: Preheat the oven to 180°C (350°F) and line a muffin tin with 4 liners.
2. **Mix wet ingredients**: In a bowl, combine grated zucchini, egg, olive oil, and maple syrup.
3. **Mix dry ingredients**: In a separate bowl, mix almond flour, cinnamon, baking powder, and sea salt.
4. **Combine and fold in walnuts**: Mix the wet ingredients into the dry ingredients and fold in the chopped walnuts.
5. **Bake**: Pour the batter into muffin liners and bake for 18-20 minutes or until a toothpick comes out clean.
6. **Cool and serve**: Let the muffins cool for a few minutes before serving.

Nutritional Facts (Per Serving):
Calories: 200 | Carbs: 15g | Protein: 6g | Fat: 15g | Sugar: 6g

Variations and Tips

For diabetics: Use a sugar-free sweetener like erythritol instead of maple syrup.
For allergies: Replace walnuts with pumpkin seeds for a nut-free version.
Flavor tip: Add a pinch of nutmeg for extra spice

Chia Seed Pudding with Mango

Prep: 5 min   Cook: N/A (Chill for 2hours)   Serves:2

Ingredients:

- 1/4 cup (40g) chia seeds
- 1 cup (240ml) almond milk (or any plant-based milk)
- 1 tbsp (15ml) maple syrup
- 1/2 tsp vanilla extract
- 1/2 cup (120g) fresh mango, diced

Instructions:

1. **Mix ingredients**: In a bowl, combine chia seeds, almond milk, maple syrup, and vanilla extract. Stir well to combine.
2. **Chill**: Refrigerate for at least 2 hours or overnight, stirring once after 30 minutes to avoid clumps.
3. **Serve with mango**: Once the pudding has thickened, top with diced mango and enjoy

Nutritional Facts (Per Serving):
Calories: 180 | Carbs: 20g | Protein: 5g | Fat: 9g | Sugar: 10g

Variations and Tips

For diabetics: Use unsweetened almond milk and reduce the amount of maple syrup or replace it with a sugar-free sweetener.
For allergies: Swap almond milk for coconut or oat milk for a nut-free version.
Flavor tip: Add a sprinkle of coconut flakes for extra texture.

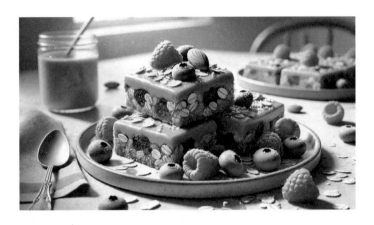

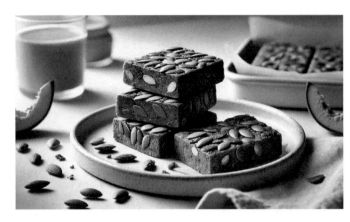

Almond Butter and Berry Oat Bars

Prep: 10 minutes   Cook: 20 minutes   Serves: 2

Ingredients:

- 1/2 cup (45g) rolled oats
- 1/4 cup (60g) almond butter
- 2 tbsp (30ml) maple syrup
- 1/4 cup (50g) fresh mixed berries (or frozen, thawed)
- 1 tbsp (15ml) coconut oil, melted
- 1/2 tsp cinnamon
- 1/4 tsp baking powder
- 1/4 tsp sea salt

Instructions:

1. **Preheat the oven**: Preheat oven to 180°C (350°F) and line a small baking dish with parchment paper.
2. **Mix wet ingredients**: In a bowl, combine almond butter, maple syrup, and coconut oil until smooth.
3. **Add dry ingredients**: Stir in oats, cinnamon, baking powder, and salt until well combined. Gently fold in the berries.
4. **Bake**: Transfer the mixture to the prepared dish and bake for 18-20 minutes until golden brown.
5. **Cool and serve**: Let the bars cool before slicing and serving.

Nutritional Facts (Per Serving):
Calories: 240 | Carbs: 20g | Protein: 6g | Fat: 16g | Sugar: 8g

Variations and Tips

For diabetics: Reduce the maple syrup or replace it with a sugar-free sweetener.
For allergies: Use sunflower seed butter instead of almond butter for a nut-free alternative.
Flavor tip: Add 1 tbsp chia seeds for extra fiber and crunch.

Pumpkin Seed Protein Bars with Cacao

Prep:10 min   Cook:N/A (Chill for 1hours)   Serves:2

Ingredients:

- 1/2 cup (75g) pumpkin seeds
- 1/4 cup (25g) cacao nibs
- 2 tbsp (30ml) coconut oil, melted
- 1 tbsp (15ml) maple syrup
- 1/4 cup (40g) protein powder (optional, plant-based for anti-inflammatory benefits)
- 1/2 tsp cinnamon
- 1/4 tsp sea salt

Instructions:

1. **Mix ingredients**: In a large bowl, combine pumpkin seeds, cacao nibs, coconut oil, maple syrup, protein powder, cinnamon, and sea salt. Stir until well combined.
2. **Shape the bars**: Transfer the mixture into a lined baking dish, pressing down firmly to form an even layer.
3. **Chill**: Refrigerate for 1 hour until the bars set.
4. **Serve**: Once set, cut into bars and enjoy as a snack or post-workout boost.

Nutritional Facts (Per Serving):
Calories: 230 | Carbs: 14g | Protein: 9g | Fat: 16g | Sugar: 6g

Variations and Tips

For diabetics: Use a sugar-free sweetener instead of maple syrup.
For allergies: Replace pumpkin seeds with sunflower seeds for a nut-free option.
Flavor tip: Add 1 tsp vanilla extract for a sweeter flavor profile.

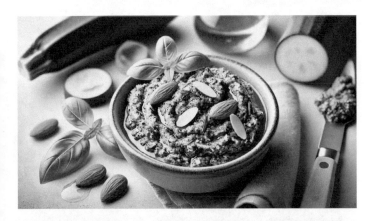

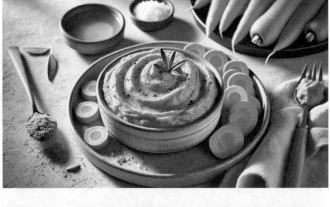

Zucchini Basil Pesto with Almonds

Prep: 10 minutes   **Cook: N/A**   **Serves: 2**

Ingredients:

- 1 medium zucchini (150g), grated
- 1/4 cup (25g) almonds
- 1/4 cup (15g) fresh basil leaves
- 1 garlic clove
- 2 tbsp (30ml) olive oil
- 1 tbsp (15ml) lemon juice
- 1/4 tsp sea salt
- 1/4 cup (30g) grated Parmesan (optional)

Instructions:

1. **Blend**: In a food processor, combine grated zucchini, almonds, basil, garlic, olive oil, lemon juice, and sea salt. Blend until smooth.
2. **Optional**: Stir in Parmesan for a richer flavor.
3. **Serve**: Use as a sauce for pasta, dip for veggies, or spread for sandwiches.

Nutritional Facts (Per Serving):
Calories: 180 | Carbs: 6g | Protein: 4g | Fat: 16g | Sugar: 2g

Variations and Tips

For diabetics: Omit the Parmesan and use nutritional yeast for a lower-fat option.
For allergies: Swap almonds for sunflower seeds for a nut-free version.
Flavor tip: Add 1 tsp of chili flakes for a spicy kick.

Pumpkin and Carrot Tahini Dip with Cumin

Prep: 10 minutes   **Cook: 20 minutes**   **Serves: 2**

Ingredients:

- 1 cup (150g) pumpkin, diced
- 1/2 cup (75g) carrots, chopped
- 2 tbsp (30g) tahini
- 1 tbsp (15ml) olive oil
- 1 tsp cumin
- 1/2 tsp sea salt
- 1 tbsp (15ml) lemon juice
- 1 garlic clove, minced

Instructions:

1. **Preheat the oven**: Preheat your oven to 180°C (350°F).
2. **Prepare the beets**: Thinly slice the beets using a mandoline or knife. Toss them with olive oil, sea salt, and black pepper.
3. **Roast the chips**: Lay the beet slices in a single layer on a baking sheet. Roast for 25-30 minutes, flipping halfway through, until crispy.
4. **Serve**: Let the beet chips cool for a few minutes before serving.

Nutritional Facts (Per Serving):
Calories: 170 | Carbs: 14g | Protein: 4g | Fat: 11g | Sugar: 4g

Variations and Tips

For diabetics: Reduce the amount of tahini or replace with Greek yogurt for lower fat and sugar content.
For allergies: Replace tahini with sunflower seed butter for a nut-free option.
Flavor tip: Add a pinch of smoked paprika for extra depth.

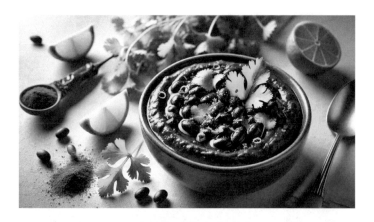

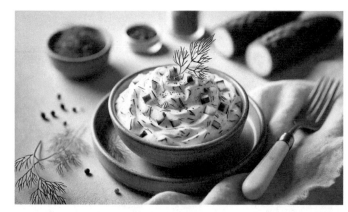

Spicy Black Bean Dip with Cilantro and Lime

Prep: 10 minutes   **Cook: N/A**   **Serves: 2**

Ingredients:

- 1 cup (240g) canned black beans, rinsed and drained
- 1 tbsp (15ml) olive oil
- 2 tbsp (30ml) lime juice
- 1 garlic clove, minced
- 1/2 tsp ground cumin
- 1/4 tsp chili powder (adjust for spice preference)
- 2 tbsp fresh cilantro, chopped
- 1/4 tsp sea salt

Instructions:

1. **Blend ingredients**: In a food processor, combine black beans, olive oil, lime juice, garlic, cumin, chili powder, and sea salt. Blend until smooth.
2. **Add cilantro**: Stir in the fresh cilantro for added flavor.
3. **Serve**: Transfer to a bowl and serve with veggie sticks or crackers.

Nutritional Facts (Per Serving):
Calories: 180 | Carbs: 22g | Protein: 6g | Fat: 7g | Sugar: 0g

Variations and Tips

For diabetics: Use a low-sodium option for canned beans and reduce the lime juice slightly.
For allergies: Replace black beans with chickpeas for an alternative legume option.
Flavor tip: Add a pinch of smoked paprika for extra depth of flavor.

Cucumber & Dill Yogurt Spread

Prep: 10 minutes   **Cook: N/A**   **Serves: 2**

Ingredients:

- 1/2 cup (120g) plain Greek yogurt
- 1/2 cucumber (75g), grated and squeezed to remove excess water
- 1 tbsp (15ml) lemon juice
- 1 garlic clove, minced
- 1 tbsp fresh dill, chopped
- 1/4 tsp sea salt
- 1/4 tsp black pepper

Instructions:

1. **Mix ingredients**: In a bowl, combine Greek yogurt, grated cucumber, lemon juice, garlic, dill, sea salt, and pepper. Stir until smooth.
2. **Serve**: Use as a spread for wraps, a dip for veggies, or a side for grilled meats.

Nutritional Facts (Per Serving):
Calories: 70 | Carbs: 5g | Protein: 6g | Fat: 2g | Sugar: 3g

Variations and Tips

For diabetics: Choose unsweetened, low-fat yogurt to control sugar and fat intake.
For allergies: Substitute Greek yogurt with a dairy-free option like coconut or almond yogurt.
Flavor tip: Add a pinch of cayenne pepper for a spicy twist.

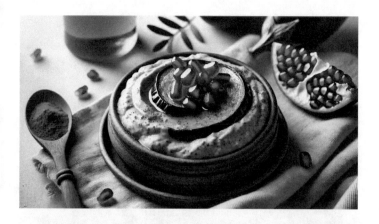

Smoky Eggplant Dip with Pomegranate

Prep: 10 minutes   **Cook: 30 minutes**   **Serves: 2**

Ingredients:

- 1 medium eggplant (200g)
- 1 tbsp (15ml) olive oil
- 2 tbsp (30g) tahini
- 1 tbsp (15ml) lemon juice
- 1 garlic clove, minced
- 1/2 tsp smoked paprika
- 2 tbsp pomegranate seeds
- 1/4 tsp sea salt

Instructions:

1. **Roast the eggplant**: Preheat the oven to 200°C (400°F). Pierce the eggplant with a fork and roast for 30 minutes until soft.
2. **Blend the dip**: Once the eggplant is cool, scoop out the flesh and blend with tahini, olive oil, lemon juice, garlic, smoked paprika, and sea salt until smooth.
3. **Serve**: Transfer to a bowl and sprinkle with pomegranate seeds. Serve with flatbread or veggie sticks.

Nutritional Facts (Per Serving):
Calories: 150 | Carbs: 12g | Protein: 3g | Fat: 10g | Sugar: 5g

Variations and Tips

For diabetics: Use less tahini and replace with Greek yogurt to lower the fat content.
For allergies: Replace tahini with sunflower seed butter for a nut-free version.
Flavor tip: Add a pinch of chili flakes for extra heat

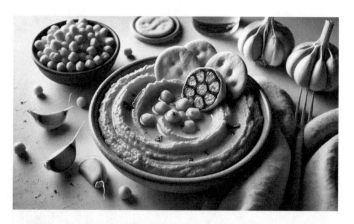

Sweet Potato & Roasted Garlic Hummus

Prep: 10 minutes   **Cook: 10 minutes**   **Serves: 2**

Ingredients:

- 1 medium sweet potato (150g), roasted and mashed
- 1/2 cup (120g) canned chickpeas, rinsed and drained
- 1 whole garlic bulb, roasted
- 2 tbsp (30ml) olive oil
- 2 tbsp (30g) tahini
- 1 tbsp (15ml) lemon juice
- 1/2 tsp ground cumin
- 1/4 tsp sea salt

Instructions:

1. **Roast the garlic**: Preheat oven to 200°C (400°F). Slice the top off the garlic bulb, drizzle with olive oil, and wrap in foil. Roast for 25 minutes.
2. **Prepare the hummus**: Blend mashed sweet potato, chickpeas, roasted garlic, olive oil, tahini, lemon juice, cumin, and sea salt until smooth.
3. **Serve**: Drizzle with extra olive oil and serve with pita or crackers.

Nutritional Facts (Per Serving):
Calories: 190 | Carbs: 24g | Protein: 4g | Fat: 9g | Sugar: 6g

Variations and Tips

For diabetics: Reduce the amount of sweet potato or chickpeas to lower the carb content.
For allergies: Replace tahini with Greek yogurt for a lighter alternative.
Flavor tip: Add a pinch of cinnamon for a sweeter, warmer flavor.

Snack Smart, Stay Healthy: Roast Up Some Veggies

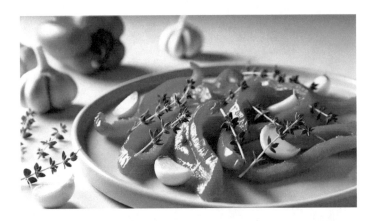

Roasted Red Peppers with Garlic and Thyme

Prep: 5 minutes   **Cook: 20 minutes**   **Serves: 2**

Ingredients:

- 2 large red bell peppers (200g)
- 1 tbsp (15ml) olive oil
- 2 garlic cloves, thinly sliced
- 1 tsp fresh thyme leaves
- 1/4 tsp sea salt
- 1/4 tsp black pepper

Instructions:

1. **Preheat oven**: Preheat to 200°C (400°F).
2. **Roast the peppers**: Slice the red peppers into thick strips, drizzle with olive oil, and toss with garlic, thyme, salt, and pepper. Spread evenly on a baking sheet.
3. **Cook**: Roast for 20 minutes until the peppers are tender and slightly charred.
4. **Serve**: Transfer to a plate and serve warm as a side dish or salad topping

Nutritional Facts (Per Serving):
Calories: 120 | Carbs: 10g | Protein: 1g | Fat: 9g | Sugar: 6g

Variations and Tips

For diabetics: Use less olive oil to reduce fat content.
For allergies: Add a splash of lemon juice for a fresh alternative to thyme.
Flavor tip: Sprinkle with a bit of smoked paprika for a deeper flavor.

Turmeric Cauliflower with Tahini Drizzle

Prep: 5 minutes   **Cook: 25 minutes**   **Serves: 2**

Ingredients:

- 1 small cauliflower (250g), cut into florets
- 1 tbsp (15ml) olive oil
- 1/2 tsp ground turmeric
- 1/4 tsp ground cumin
- 2 tbsp (30g) tahini
- 1 tbsp (15ml) lemon juice
- 1 garlic clove, minced
- 1/4 tsp sea salt

Instructions:

1. **Preheat oven**: Preheat to 200°C (400°F).
2. **Roast the cauliflower**: Toss cauliflower florets with olive oil, turmeric, cumin, and sea salt. Spread on a baking sheet and roast for 25 minutes until golden and crispy.
3. **Make the tahini drizzle**: In a small bowl, mix tahini, lemon juice, garlic, and a splash of water until smooth.
4. **Serve**: Drizzle the tahini sauce over the roasted cauliflower and enjoy.

Nutritional Facts (Per Serving):
Calories: 150 | Carbs: 12g | Protein: 4g | Fat: 11g | Sugar: 3g

Variations and Tips

For diabetics: Use less tahini to reduce fat content and calories.
For allergies: Replace tahini with sunflower seed butter for a nut-free version.
Flavor tip: Add a sprinkle of red pepper flakes for extra heat.

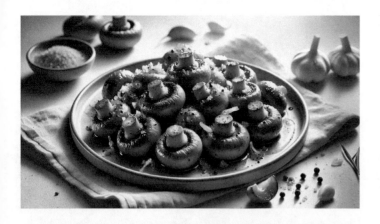

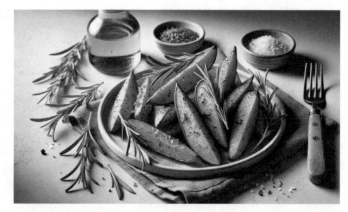

Ginger Soy Roasted Mushrooms

Prep: 10 minutes   Cook: 20 minutes   Serves: 2

Ingredients:

- 200g mushrooms (e.g., cremini or button), cleaned and halved
- 1 tbsp (15ml) soy sauce (use low-sodium for a healthier option)
- 1 tbsp (15ml) olive oil
- 1 tsp fresh ginger, grated
- 1 garlic clove, minced
- 1/2 tsp sesame oil (optional)
- 1/4 tsp black pepper

Instructions:

1. **Preheat oven**: Preheat to 200°C (400°F).
2. **Marinate the mushrooms**: In a bowl, mix soy sauce, olive oil, ginger, garlic, sesame oil (if using), and black pepper. Toss the mushrooms in the mixture until coated.
3. **Roast**: Spread the mushrooms on a baking sheet and roast for 20 minutes, stirring halfway through, until golden and tender.
4. **Serve**: Serve warm as a side or a topping for grains or salads.

Nutritional Facts (Per Serving):
Calories: 110 | Carbs: 5g | Protein: 3g | Fat: 9g | Sugar: 2g

Variations and Tips

For diabetics: Use a low-sodium soy sauce to reduce sodium intake.
For allergies: Replace soy sauce with tamari for a gluten-free option.
Flavor tip: Add a sprinkle of chili flakes for a spicy kick.

Rosemary Sweet Potato Wedges with Olive Oil

Prep: 5 minutes   Cook: 25 minutes   Serves: 2

Ingredients:

- 2 medium sweet potatoes (300g), cut into wedges
- 1 tbsp (15ml) olive oil
- 1 tsp fresh rosemary, chopped
- 1/4 tsp sea salt
- 1/4 tsp black pepper

Instructions:

1. **Preheat oven**: Preheat to 200°C (400°F).
2. **Season the potatoes**: Toss sweet potato wedges with olive oil, rosemary, salt, and pepper until well coated.
3. **Roast**: Spread the wedges on a baking sheet in a single layer and roast for 25 minutes, flipping halfway, until golden and crispy.
4. **Serve**: Serve as a side or enjoy as a healthy snack.

Nutritional Facts (Per Serving):
Calories: 180 | Carbs: 30g | Protein: 2g | Fat: 7g | Sugar: 6g

Variations and Tips

For diabetics: Reduce the portion size of sweet potatoes to control carbohydrate intake.
For allergies: Replace olive oil with avocado oil for a different flavor.
Flavor tip: Add a sprinkle of smoked paprika for an extra layer of flavor.

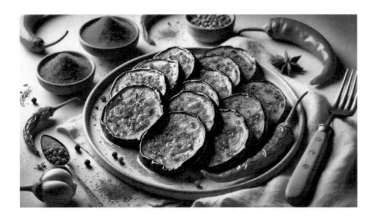

Spicy Eggplant Slices with Smoked Paprika

Prep: 5 minutes   Cook: 20 minutes   Serves: 2

Ingredients:

- 1 medium eggplant (250g), sliced into rounds
- 1 tbsp (15ml) olive oil
- 1 tsp smoked paprika
- 1/2 tsp ground cumin
- 1/4 tsp sea salt
- 1/4 tsp black pepper
- 1/4 tsp red chili flakes (optional for extra spice)

Instructions:

1. **Preheat oven**: Preheat to 200°C (400°F).
2. **Season the eggplant**: Toss eggplant slices with olive oil, smoked paprika, cumin, sea salt, black pepper, and chili flakes.
3. **Roast**: Arrange the eggplant slices on a baking sheet and roast for 20 minutes, flipping halfway through, until golden and tender.
4. **Serve**: Serve warm as a side dish or as a topping for grains or salads.

Nutritional Facts (Per Serving):
Calories: 120 | Carbs: 10g | Protein: 2g | Fat: 8g | Sugar: 4g

Variations and Tips

For diabetics: Reduce the amount of oil to lower fat content.
For allergies: Substitute olive oil with avocado oil for a nut-free alternative.
Flavor tip: Add a drizzle of tahini for a creamier texture.

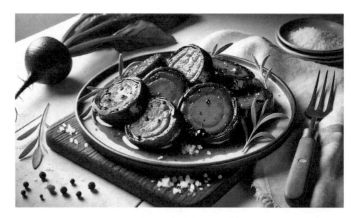

Caramelized Beets with Balsamic Vinegar

Prep: 5 minutes   Cook: 30 minutes   Serves: 2

Ingredients:

- 2 medium beets (200g), peeled and sliced
- 1 tbsp (15ml) olive oil
- 1 tbsp (15ml) balsamic vinegar
- 1 tsp honey or maple syrup
- 1/4 tsp sea salt
- 1/4 tsp black pepper

Instructions:

1. **Preheat oven**: Preheat to 200°C (400°F).
2. **Caramelize the beets**: Toss beet slices with olive oil, balsamic vinegar, honey or maple syrup, sea salt, and black pepper.
3. **Roast**: Spread the beets evenly on a baking sheet and roast for 30 minutes, flipping halfway through, until tender and caramelized.
4. **Serve**: Serve warm as a side dish or add to salads.

Nutritional Facts (Per Serving):
Calories: 140 | Carbs: 18g | Protein: 2g | Fat: 7g | Sugar: 12g

Variations and Tips

For diabetics: Omit the honey or use a sugar substitute to reduce sugar content.
For allergies: Replace olive oil with coconut oil for a different flavor.
Flavor tip: Garnish with fresh herbs like thyme or parsley for a refreshing finish.

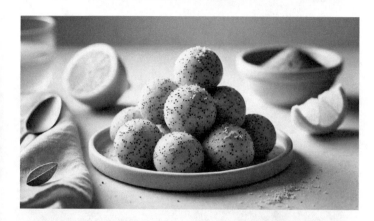

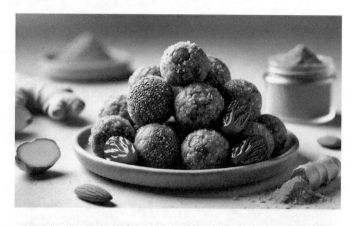

Lemon Poppy Seed Protein Bites

Prep: 10 minutes	Cook: N/A	Serves: 2

Ingredients:

- 1/2 cup (120g) almond flour
- 1 tbsp (15ml) lemon juice
- 1 tbsp (15g) poppy seeds
- 2 tbsp (30g) honey or maple syrup
- 1 tbsp (15ml) coconut oil, melted
- 1 scoop (30g) vanilla protein powder (optional for extra protein)
- 1/4 tsp lemon zest
- 1/4 tsp sea salt

Instructions:

1. **Mix the ingredients**: In a bowl, combine almond flour, poppy seeds, protein powder (if using), lemon juice, honey or maple syrup, coconut oil, lemon zest, and salt. Stir until well combined.
2. **Shape into bites**: Roll the mixture into small bite-sized balls and refrigerate for at least 30 minutes until firm.
3. **Serve**: Enjoy as a snack or quick energy boost.

Nutritional Facts (Per Serving):
Calories: 150 | Carbs: 10g | Protein: 8g | Fat: 11g | Sugar: 6g

Variations and Tips

For diabetics: Use a sugar-free syrup or honey substitute to reduce sugar content.
For allergies: Replace almond flour with oat flour for a nut-free version.
Flavor tip: Add a pinch of vanilla extract for extra depth of flavor.

Ginger-Turmeric Power Bites with Dates

Prep: 10 minutes	Cook: N/A	Serves: 2

Ingredients:

- 1/2 cup (100g) pitted dates
- 1/4 cup (60g) almonds
- 1/2 tsp ground turmeric
- 1/2 tsp ground ginger
- 1 tbsp (15g) chia seeds
- 1 tbsp (15ml) coconut oil, melted

Instructions:

1. **Blend ingredients**: In a food processor, combine dates, almonds, turmeric, ginger, chia seeds, and coconut oil. Blend until it forms a sticky, well-combined mixture.
2. **Form bites**: Shape the mixture into bite-sized balls and refrigerate for 20 minutes until firm.
3. **Serve**: Enjoy as a nutritious snack for an energy boost.

Nutritional Facts (Per Serving):
Calories: 210 | Carbs:25g | Protein: 5g | Fat:10g | Sugar: 16g

Variations and Tips

For diabetics: Limit the amount of dates and balance with more nuts or seeds.
For allergies: Use pumpkin seeds instead of almonds for a nut-free option.
Flavor tip: Add a pinch of black pepper to enhance the absorption of turmeric.

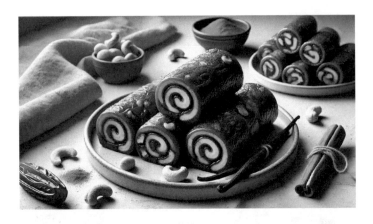

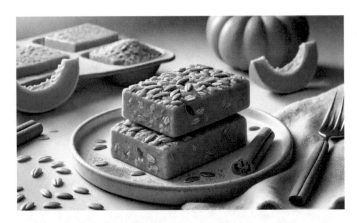

Cashew-Cinnamon Date Rolls with a Hint of Vanilla

Prep: 10 minutes   **Cook: N/A**   **Serves: 2**

Ingredients:

- 1/2 cup (120g) cashews
- 1/2 cup (100g) pitted dates
- 1/2 tsp cinnamon
- 1/2 tsp vanilla extract
- 1 tbsp (15ml) coconut oil, melted
- Pinch of sea salt

Instructions:

1. **Blend ingredients**: In a food processor, combine cashews, dates, cinnamon, vanilla extract, coconut oil, and sea salt. Process until the mixture becomes sticky and holds together.
2. **Form rolls**: Roll the mixture into small log shapes or balls, and refrigerate for 20 minutes until firm.
3. **Serve**: Enjoy as a snack or dessert.

Nutritional Facts (Per Serving):
Calories: 220 | Carbs: 30g | Protein: 4g | Fat: 11g | Sugar: 20g

Variations and Tips

For diabetics: Reduce dates and replace with a lower glycemic fruit like dried apricots.
For allergies: Substitute cashews with sunflower seeds for a nut-free option.
Flavor tip: Add a pinch of nutmeg for an extra warm spice flavor.

Pumpkin Spice Protein Bars with Flaxseeds

Prep: 10 minutes   **Cook: N/A**   **Serves: 2**

Ingredients:

- 1/2 cup (120g) canned pumpkin puree
- 1/2 cup (50g) rolled oats
- 1 tbsp (15g) ground flaxseeds
- 1 tbsp (15ml) maple syrup
- 1 tbsp (15g) almond butter
- 1 scoop (30g) vanilla protein powder
- 1 tsp pumpkin spice
- 1/4 tsp cinnamon
- 1/4 tsp sea salt

Instructions:

1. **Combine ingredients**: In a large bowl, mix together pumpkin puree, rolled oats, flaxseeds, maple syrup, almond butter, protein powder, pumpkin spice, cinnamon, and sea salt until fully combined.
2. **Form into bars**: Press the mixture into a small baking dish lined with parchment paper and refrigerate for at least 1 hour until firm.
3. **Slice and serve**: Once set, slice into bars and enjoy as a healthy snack.

Nutritional Facts (Per Serving):
Calories: 180 | Carbs: 22g | Protein: 10g | Fat: 8g | Sugar: 7g

Variations and Tips

For diabetics: Reduce the maple syrup or replace it with a sugar-free alternative.
For allergies: Substitute almond butter with sunflower seed butter for a nut-free version.
Flavor tip: Add a handful of chopped walnuts or pecans for extra crunch.

CHAPTER 4: KEEP GOING STRONG

Key Takeaways for Lifelong Wellness

As you continue your journey toward a healthier, anti-inflammatory lifestyle, it's important to remember that this is not a short-term fix. It's a lifelong commitment to improving your health, managing inflammation, and achieving overall wellness. Staying consistent, flexible, and focused on your long-term goals is essential.

There are several key principles to remember as you move forward. First, **balance is key**. Eating a variety of anti-inflammatory foods rich in nutrients is fundamental to long-term health. Don't be afraid to try new foods, flavors, and recipes that align with your goals.

Second, **self-care goes beyond just food**. A healthy lifestyle includes proper sleep, stress management, and regular physical activity. These factors play a significant role in reducing inflammation and maintaining wellness. Incorporate movement you enjoy, whether it's walking, yoga, or strength training—whatever helps you feel your best.

Finally, **stay flexible**. Life changes, and your needs will evolve over time. Be willing to adjust your diet and lifestyle based on what your body tells you. The anti-inflammatory approach is adaptable, whether you're dealing with new health challenges, lifestyle shifts, or simply want to try something different.

Review and Adjust Your Plan

As you progress through your anti-inflammatory journey, it's essential to regularly review and adjust your plan. This is not a one-size-fits-all approach—each person's body responds differently to dietary changes. You'll want to periodically assess how you're feeling, both physically and mentally, and make necessary adjustments to ensure the plan is working optimally for you.

Start by identifying any changes in your symptoms. Are you noticing a decrease in inflammation or improvements in energy levels? Maybe your digestion has improved, or you're sleeping better. On the other hand, you might discover that certain foods aren't having the desired effect, or they may even be causing new issues. Take note of these and be willing to adapt your meal choices to better suit your needs.

For instance, if a certain ingredient feels heavy on your stomach, like legumes, consider replacing them with easier-to-digest alternatives, such as sweet potatoes or quinoa. Similarly, if your goal is to reduce joint pain and you haven't seen significant improvement, you might want to increase the intake of omega-3-rich foods like salmon and walnuts. Adjustments like these can be small but impactful, keeping you on track toward better health.

Track Your Progress

Tracking your progress is a crucial step in any dietary plan. It gives you insight into what's working and what needs adjustment. Consider keeping a food journal, noting not only what you eat but also how you feel afterward. Track any changes in inflammation, energy levels, mood, digestion, and even how well you're sleeping.

If you've had a stressful week and notice more inflammation, it could be related to food choices or external factors like stress. By recognizing patterns, you'll be able to adjust your diet accordingly. Maybe after a week of lower energy levels, you find that adding more nutrient-dense, anti-inflammatory snacks like pumpkin seeds or turmeric lattes helps get you back on track. Keeping records ensures that you're not guessing when it comes to your health.

Make Long-Term Adjustments

Once you've been on this plan for a while, you'll start to notice which foods work best for your body and which might not. As your health improves, your body's needs may also change. That's why it's important to be flexible and make long-term adjustments to continue supporting your overall wellness.

For example, if you've initially avoided nightshades like tomatoes or eggplants to reduce inflammation and notice significant improvement, you might experiment with slowly reintroducing them to see how your body responds. Alternatively, if you're feeling more energized, you might shift your focus to foods that support long-term vitality, such as incorporating more antioxidants and fiber-rich vegetables like kale and berries.

It's also vital to adjust your plan based on your lifestyle. If you're preparing for a more active phase in life, like training for a race or starting a new fitness routine, your body will require additional support through increased protein or more energy-sustaining meals. This might involve adding extra servings of lean protein like chicken or plant-based sources like chickpeas, depending on your dietary preferences.

By regularly reviewing your plan, tracking your progress, and making long-term adjustments, you'll create a sustainable anti-inflammatory lifestyle that enhances your overall health and well-being. This flexible approach ensures that your diet evolves with you, meeting your body's needs as they change.

Stay on Track for Good

Maintaining a healthy anti-inflammatory lifestyle isn't about perfection—it's about consistency. By sticking to your routine, navigating social situations confidently, and adapting to life's inevitable changes, you can stay on track for the long term without feeling overwhelmed. Here's how you can do it effectively.

Stick to Your Routine

One of the most critical aspects of staying on track with your anti-inflammatory diet is establishing a routine that works for you and sticking to it. This doesn't mean being rigid, but rather finding balance in your daily choices. When healthy eating becomes part of your routine, it feels less like a chore and more like a natural part of your day.

Meal prep can play a big role in keeping you on track. Dedicate time each week to prepare meals and snacks that align with your diet. By having healthy, anti-inflammatory options readily available, you'll be less likely to stray from your plan. If mornings are busy, prepare breakfast the night before—overnight oats or chia seed pudding are great options. When your routine is in place, it removes the guesswork and keeps you focused on your goals.

Remember, it's okay to be flexible. Life happens. If you miss a meal or have an unexpected indulgence, don't let it derail your progress. Get back on track with your next meal, and remind yourself that consistency over time matters more than occasional slip-ups.

Navigate Social Situations

Social events can often feel like a challenge when you're committed to a specific diet, especially one focused on reducing inflammation. Whether it's dining out with friends or attending a family gathering, it's important to feel empowered in your choices without feeling deprived.

When eating out, don't hesitate to ask for modifications. Many restaurants are more than willing to accommodate dietary preferences. Opt for grilled proteins, salads, and vegetable-based dishes. For example, swap out starchy sides for a simple salad or steamed vegetables. You can also check the menu in advance to plan your meal ahead of time.

In situations where food is provided, like parties or gatherings, consider bringing a dish that aligns with your diet. This ensures you have something nutritious to enjoy while sharing your healthy choices with others. And if you indulge in something outside your typical diet, remember to enjoy it without guilt and return to your routine the next day. Maintaining a positive mindset about food is essential for long-term success.

Adapt to Life's Changes

Life is unpredictable, and your routine will inevitably be interrupted at times—whether it's a busy workweek, travel, or a personal challenge. Adapting your anti-inflammatory diet to life's changes ensures that your healthy habits remain sustainable, no matter what comes your way.

For busy periods, keep your meals simple. Lean on easy, nutrient-dense staples like salads, smoothies, or grain bowls that can be prepared quickly. Batch cooking can also help—freeze individual portions of soups or stews so you always have something ready when time is tight.

When traveling, pack snacks like nuts, seeds, or dried fruits that travel well and keep you energized. Look for local restaurants or grocery stores that offer fresh, whole food options. If your routine is interrupted for an extended period, remember that your anti-inflammatory journey is a marathon, not a sprint. Focus on small, manageable changes and get back into your routine as soon as you can.

Conclusion

Staying on track with an anti-inflammatory diet is about developing sustainable habits that work for your lifestyle. By sticking to a flexible routine, navigating social situations with confidence, and adapting to life's inevitable changes, you can maintain the benefits of this healthy lifestyle long term. It's not about perfection—it's about creating a balanced approach to nutrition that supports your overall well-being.

Your journey doesn't have to be perfect. It's important to celebrate the small victories, whether it's trying a new recipe, making better food choices, or noticing improvements in your energy and overall well-being. Every step forward counts

Acknowledgments

Dear Reader,

I hope this book has been a helpful guide on your journey toward better health and well-being. If these recipes and insights have brought even a small spark of inspiration or made a positive impact on your life, I would be incredibly grateful if you could share your thoughts.

Your reviews not only help others discover how these simple steps can lead to lasting change, but they also give me the motivation to continue

creating content that supports you in your wellness journey. Whether it's a favorite recipe, a breakthrough moment, or simply the joy of discovering new, healthier habits — your feedback matters.

Thank you for being a part of this journey. Your success is my inspiration, and your voice helps this community grow stronger.

With heartfelt gratitude, Iris Mayfie

Made in the USA
Columbia, SC
02 January 2025

50997206R00041